D0594013

EARLY WARNING

MEDICAL ETHICS SERIES

David H. Smith and Robert M. Veatch, Editors

Norman L. Cantor. *Advance Directives and the Pursuit of Death with Dignity*

Norman L. Cantor. *Legal Frontiers of Death and Dying*

Arthur L. Caplan. *Am I My Brother's Keeper? The Ethical Frontiers of Biomedicine*

Arthur L. Caplan. *If I Were a Rich Man Could I Buy a Pancreas? And Other Essays on the Ethics of Health Care*

James F. Childress. *Practical Reasoning in Bioethics: Principles, Metaphors, and Analogies*

Cynthia B. Cohen, ed. *Casebook on the Termination of Life-Sustaining Treatment and the Care of the Dying*

Cynthia B. Cohen, ed. *New Ways of Making Babies: The Case of Egg Donation*

Roger B. Dworkin. *Limits: The Role of the Law in Bioethical Decision Making*

Larry Gostin, ed. *Surrogate Motherhood: Politics and Privacy*

Christine Grady. *The Search for an AIDS Vaccine: Ethical Issues in the Development and Testing of a Preventive HIV Vaccine*

A Report by the Hastings Center. *Guidelines on the Termination of Life-Sustaining Treatment and the Care of the Dying*

Paul Lauritzen. *Pursuing Parenthood: Ethical Issues in Assisted Reproduction*

Joanne Lynn, M.D., ed. *By No Extraordinary Means: The Choice to Forgo Life-Sustaining Food and Water, Expanded Edition*

William F. May. *The Patient's Ordeal*

Richard W. Momeyer. *Confronting Death*

Thomas H. Murray, Mark A. Rothstein, and Robert F. Murray, Jr., eds. *The Human Genome Project and the Future of Health Care*

S. Kay Toombs, David Barnard, and Ronald Carson, eds. *Chronic Illness: From Experience to Policy*

Robert M. Veatch. *The Patient as Partner: A Theory of Human-Experimentation Ethics*

Robert M. Veatch. *The Patient-Physician Relation: The Patient as Partner, Part 2*

Robert F. Weir, ed. *Physician-Assisted Suicide*

Early Warning

CASES AND ETHICAL GUIDANCE FOR PRESYMPTOMATIC TESTING IN GENETIC DISEASES

David H. Smith, Kimberly A. Quaid,
Roger B. Dworkin, Gregory P. Gramelspacher,
Judith A. Granbois, and Gail H. Vance

INDIANA UNIVERSITY PRESS
Bloomington and Indianapolis

MIDDLEBURY COLLEGE LIBRARY

This book is a publication of

Indiana University Press
601 North Morton Street
Bloomington, Indiana 47404-3797 USA

www.indiana.edu/~iupress

Telephone orders   800-842-6796
Fax orders   812-855-7931
Orders by e-mail   iuporder@indiana.edu

© 1998 by Indiana University Press

All rights reserved

No part of this book may be reproduced or utilized in any
form or by any means, electronic or mechanical, including
photocopying and recording, or by any information storage
and retrieval system, without permission in writing from the
publisher. The Association of American University Presses'
Resolution on Permissions constitutes the only exception
to this prohibition.

The paper used in this publication meets the minimum
requirements of American National Standard for
Information Sciences—Permanence of Paper for Printed
Library Materials, ANSI Z39.48-1984.

Manufactured in the United States of America

Library of Congress Cataloging-in-Publication Data

Early warning : cases and ethical guidance for presymptomatic testing
   in genetic diseases / David H. Smith . . . [et al.].
      p.   cm. — (Medical ethics series)
   Includes bibliographical references and index.
   ISBN 0-253-33401-2 (cl : alk. paper)
      1. Genetic disorders—Diagnosis—Moral and ethical aspects.
   2. Genetic disorders—Diagnosis—Case studies.   I. Series.
   [DNLM: 1. Huntington's Disease—diagnosis case studies.
   2. Huntington's Disease—genetics.   3. Hereditary Diseases—
   diagnosis case studies.   4. Ethics, Medical.   5. Genetic Screening
   case studies.   6. Genetic Counseling. WL 390 E12 1998]
   RB155.6.E27   1998
   616'.042—dc21
   DNLM/DLC
   for Library of Congress   98-3978

1   2   3   4   5   03   02   01   00   99   98

Contents

Acknowledgments   *vii*

Introduction   *1*

Cases

Case 1   Paul and Michael   *21*

Case 2   Father and Son   *26*

Case 3   Sarah   *29*

Case 4   Ann and Jack   *33*

Case 5   Carol   *39*

Case 6   Kirsten and David   *42*

Case 7   Robert   *46*

Case 8   Mr. H.   *50*

Case 9   Natalie   *53*

Case 10   Mary Ann   *58*

Case 11   Maurice   *62*

Case 12   Mr. L.   *68*

Case 13   Mr. Crawford   *72*

Case 14   Mr. and Mrs. Anderson   *76*

Case 15   Jimmy   *80*

Case 16   Harriet   *84*

Case 17   Charley   *87*

Case 18   Mr. and Mrs. B.   *90*

Case 19   Julie   *94*

Case 20   Barbara   *98*

Case 21   Doug   *102*

Case 22   Uncle Lee   *106*

Case 23   Emily   *109*

Case 24   Mrs. K.   *113*

Case 25 Ruth   *115*

Case 26 Jackie   *117*

Case 27 Aunt Mary   *121*

Case 28 Scott   *123*

Case 29 Mrs. Sawyer   *126*

Guidelines and Commentary

Guideline I Skilled Professional Counseling   *131*

Guideline II Appropriate Information   *137*

Guideline III Pre- and Posttest Counseling   *139*

Guideline IV Protocols   *142*

Guideline V Confidentiality   *144*

Guideline VI Refusing or Postponing Testing   *149*

Guideline VII Freedom to Reject Disclosure   *151*

Guideline VIII Others' Preference Not to Know   *155*

Guideline IX Possible Future Uses of Information   *158*

Guideline X Reproductive Choices   *161*

Guideline XI Testing Children   *163*

Glossary   *167*

References   *171*

Contributors   *183*

Index   *185*

Acknowledgments

THIS PROJECT OF ongoing discussion was made possible by funding from the Ethical, Legal and Social Implications (ELSI) branch of the National Center for Human Genome Research (Grant Number R01 00538). Our interdisciplinary working group comprised six members, evenly divided between the Indianapolis and Bloomington campuses of Indiana University. Individually, we are trained in ethics, law, medicine, medical genetics, psychology, and communication. We are a diverse group that brought several kinds of expertise to the table; we have worked together on this project for more than three years. Our greatest debts are to each other and to ELSI.

Planning the project was an intensive and extensive process. We were helped substantially along the way, notably by Peter Cherbas, IU Professor of Biology, who met with, challenged, instructed, and cajoled us for years.

Once funded, we spent the first two years of the project collecting the twenty-nine cases that constitute the body of this book and working out our stands on the issues they presented. This process entailed meeting at approximately two-week intervals, writing repeated drafts, experiencing more than one change of mind, airing frequent amicable disagreements. Two groups of consultants reviewed our developing product each year; in the third year we took sample cases on the road and visited several centers to explore their reactions. During this final year, we drafted and revised our guidelines.

Through the project, our helpers and conversation partners included first the senior consultants to the project, who met with us each May, read our work in progress, and offered enormously insightful and helpful suggestions. They are Robert Burt, Southmayd Professor of Law, Yale Law School; P. Michael Conneally, Distinguished Professor of Medical and Molecular Genetics and of Neurology, Indiana University; Thomas H. Murray, Professor and Director, Center for Biomedical Ethics, Case Western Reserve University School of Medicine; and Madison Powers, Senior Research Scholar, Kennedy Institute of Ethics, Georgetown University. Our group experienced a keen sense of regret in May of 1996, when we realized that we were meeting with them for the last time.

We profited from the experience and wisdom of Marguerite Chapman, Associate Professor of Law, The University of Tulsa College of Law;

Dorene S. Markel, Assistant Director, General Clinical Research Center, University of Michigan; and Barbara B. Smith, former Patient Services Director, Kidney Association of Oregon, Inc. They guided us through the literature, provided cases, and helped us grasp the nuances of the issues we were addressing.

We shared our case analyses in progress with a number of professional counselors and members of families at risk for genetic disease, who graciously offered their firsthand experience with late-onset genetic disorders and provided us with a vital reality check. We thank Robin Bennett, Michael Burgess, Tom Caldwell, Catherine V. Hayes, Audrey Heimler, Jill Johnson, David K. Shea, Judy Sinsheimer, Vickie Venne, and Alice Wexler.

Several researchers and other professionals gave us cases, information, and insight. We thank Dr. Michael Hayden of Vancouver, B.C., and his colleagues Sandi Wiggins, Shelin Adam, and Maurice Bloch; Dr. Richard H. Myers of Boston University School of Medicine; Drs. Jason Brandt and Ann Marie Codori of the Johns Hopkins School of Medicine; John A. Phillips, M.D.; Cindy L. Vnencak-Jones, Ph.D.; Vickie Hannig; Ellen Wright-Clayton, M.D., J.D., all of the Division of Genetics at Vanderbilt University Medical Center; Digmaber F. Borgaonker, Ph.D., Medical Center of Delaware Cytogenetics Lab; Suzanne Cassidy, Clinical Director, Center for Human Genetics, Case Western Reserve University School of Medicine; Nancy Wexler; and Carol Isaacson Barash.

At the end of the day, our book may be an illustration of what can be hoped for from serious and sustained interdisciplinary discussion. For better or worse, it lacks the distinctive author's hand of a single individual. None of us, asked to take on the task alone, would have come up with anything like it. Instead, we have a distillation of years of thought and discussion and some formulations that reflect substantial breadth of experience. We hope it will be helpful.

EARLY WARNING

Introduction

Paul, a healthy twenty-five-year-old man, contacts a testing center to request testing for Huntington disease (HD). Paul has an identical twin brother, Michael, who does not wish to have the predictive test.

Robert, the father of two young adult daughters, requests predictive genetic testing for autosomal dominant polycystic kidney disease (ADPKD). Robert's test results reveal that he does carry the gene for ADPKD. However, he refuses to inform his daughters, both of whom plan to have children soon, about his test results.

Kirsten is a twenty-nine-year-old woman whose husband, David, is at 50 percent risk for HD. She has discovered that she is six weeks pregnant, and she wants to have the fetus tested for the HD mutation. David is undecided about whether he wants the predictive test for himself. Kirsten, however, feels very strongly that she does not want their child to be at any risk for HD. Now that the technology is available, she wants to use it to enable her to decide whether to continue the pregnancy.

This book explores the complexity of life in an age of expanding genetic knowledge. Its specific focus is presymptomatic testing for late-onset, autosomal dominant genetic diseases, but the implications are much broader. During the past twenty years, knowledge about human genetics has increased at an exponential rate. Genetic information has the potential to contribute to major improvements in the health of individuals, groups, and societies. It may enable individuals to avoid illness through early intervention and, potentially, gene therapy. It can affect reproductive decisions by providing couples with information that will help them to avoid unwanted pregnancies or will give them the courage to have children.

Like all progress, however, this new knowledge brings problems in its wake. For many people at risk for a genetic disorder, the question of whether to pursue genetic testing is particularly troubling. The possibility of learning that one is not at high risk for breast cancer or Huntington disease must be tempered by the prospect that one must live with the opposite result. Genetic knowledge may be used as a basis for unwarranted discrimination or manipulation. If one decides to be tested, someone else—a child or parent or sibling—may be required to submit to examinations, give blood samples, and possibly run the risk of learning something he or she does not wish to know.

Persons who provide genetic counseling find themselves informing and advising persons such as Paul or Robert or Kirsten—persons who are at risk for genetic disease. They must tread their way carefully through a maze created by the potential promise—and the potential pitfalls—of genetic testing. We hope that this book will provide helpful guidance for those providing genetic counseling and testing as they struggle with these issues.

We are not the first persons to address the questions of whether to test, when to test, what to tell, and whom to tell. A considerable literature addresses the issues that confront persons providing genetic counseling. Some commentary takes the form of case studies, often informed by a particular moral paradigm. Various commissions and organizations have proposed sets of guidelines based on the professional experience of their membership and the life experience of those at risk for genetic disorders and their families. (See IHA/WFN 1990, 1994 and Huntington's Disease Society of America 1989, 1994.) Other individuals and groups have made important proposals, and we cite many of them in the text and in our bibliography.

Our approach is distinguishable from much of the prior work by the close connection we sustain between case discussion and limited generalization. Our proposals are rooted in the discussion of twenty-nine specific cases. We suggest some general guidelines that may follow from our resolution of the cases, but those guidelines are of little value apart from the case discussions that precede them. We believe that the process of guideline formation is dependent on case analysis, and any statement of general guidelines must follow from concrete, practical discussion of specific situations.

We hold these beliefs because the one certainty with new genetic knowledge is uncertainty. The issues with which we wrestle in this book are new, however much they may embody perennial human problems and concerns. The stakes for individuals at risk for genetic disease are high, but—although our technical knowledge is expanding rapidly—our fund of moral wisdom and our level of social consensus are low. In these circumstances, it seems most appropriate to adopt a stance of moral modesty and a style in which the dominant tone is inquiry and deliberation, rather than the enunciation of a crisp verdict. We think the place to begin is with the conflicts and uncertainties that confront counselors and consultands; any guidelines that may be drawn should be clearly and explicitly connected to those conflicts and to uncertainties that may be unresolvable.

Much writing on medical ethics begins with the development of a general set of principles, often derived from the work of great contemporary or classical philosophers. Those principles then shape and structure the way medical ethics problems are perceived, presented, and resolved. This approach captures something profound: The categories we use to interpret the world determine what constitutes a problem for us. Someone unaware of the importance of freedom or justice, for example, will not notice their absence in a human drama. Thus, presenting one's fundamental moral principles "up front" has the great advantage of candor and fair dealing. Neutral as he or she may be on the merits of the case at the outset, the moralist has taken a public stand on the perspective from which it will be approached. Moreover, the distinctive perspective sheds light and forces consideration of problems that may have been swept under the rug.

In our view, however, this method is insufficient as a way of addressing emerging issues in biomedical ethics. First, it is obvious that abstract principles are often unnecessary for the resolution of real dilemmas. Practical reasoning may lead to the sound and morally unproblematic resolution of real disputes without anybody being able to articulate the controlling principles for that resolution in advance. Given this fact, appeals to abstract principle can amount to changing the subject and moving the terms of argument into terrain where nuance and qualification are ignored. Effective debating skills may displace sensitive perceptions. Moreover, the alternative to beginning with principles need not be a pure situationalism. Studying case resolutions may lead to recognition of generalizable principles.

Second, beginning with a clear set of principles or even a single master principle may—although logically it need not—provide a rationale for spending insufficient time listening and understanding. Without a process of dialogue and discussion, problems arise from the inevitable limits of anyone's perspective on what "the issues" are. Reaching some level of agreement on the definition of the issues—let alone their resolution—is a time-consuming task and one that requires much more effort than many writers on ethics will acknowledge. A more inductive approach maximizes the opportunity to make ethical distinctions based on subtle factual differences among cases and minimizes the risks of dogmatism. The method adopted by the Anglo-American common law, it facilitates painting with a fine brush.

What is needed is a process that will foster listening and understanding. We have seen that tried on a national level with a series of highly visible national commissions, but those commissions have their own distinctive limitations of time, political pressure, and dependence on staff. Immodestly perhaps, we felt that if an interdisciplinary group were forced to listen to the voices heard in these cases—and to each other's voices—we could stretch our own imaginations and see more facets of problems than the lens of any single moral perspective would reveal.

To be sure, some losses are inherent in the process of reaching interdisciplinary consensus, and, as our minority opinions show, we did not always arrive at that goal. We do not contend that a dialogic process is necessarily self-correcting: Group discussion can move away from an important individual insight. But with new situations everyone is struggling to understand, it is highly unlikely that any single perspective will prove adequate. We built that conviction into our method.

If we were to begin with cases, we had to decide which histories or narratives would constitute a case. We had two practical criteria for case selection. First, we wanted *actual* cases that presented genetic counseling challenges. We sought cases in which family members might be subjected to pressure or coercion, difficult reproductive decisions must be confronted, or unstable but competent consultands sought testing. We wanted histories that really raised a problem for someone involved.

Second, we needed access to factual information. In order to understand the full complexities of real situations, we wanted enough detail to offer "thick description." We anticipated that our discussions with other testing centers would provide adequate data consistent with the need to safeguard the privacy of patients and families at risk.

In the event, many of our cases are pretty thin. They do not provide extensive descriptions of the consultands or their circumstances, for several reasons. We did not have and could not get information on consultands' ethnic or racial backgrounds, nor do we have reliable information about socioeconomic class. We do not know about their religious preferences or educational level or their employment status and the particular stresses and strains that status may entail. We have had to make the best of the available information.

However, even if we had had access to more detail, two other problems would surface. First, the amount of potentially relevant information that could go into the description of any case is virtually endless. In her recent book, *Mapping Fate*, Alice Wexler takes thousands of words to describe her family and its struggle with HD, including issues of testing, and she sees the issues "only" from the point of view of one participant in the drama (Wexler 1995). To describe fully the human reality of any of the situations that we compress into a few paragraphs would require great discernment; as a practical matter, it would also limit the number of cases that could be considered and the number of persons, many of them busy professionals, who could be expected to read them. If we were going to cover multiple cases, raising diverse issues, narratives had to be compressed, and details had to be selected.

Second, we have obvious moral responsibilities of confidentiality to the persons whose circumstances are reported in these pages. The more detail presented, the greater the risk to confidentiality. Sometimes the facts of a particular situation are so distinctive that even to state the situation exposes the consultand to inadvertent disclosure. To forestall that problem, we have used our discretion to change identifying details in a very few cases.

We do not advance these considerations in an attempt to rebut criticisms that our case presentations are too sparse and abstract; we wish they could be otherwise. There is a real place for more focused and ethnographically detailed studies of consultands in the genetic counseling situation. But we have thought it important to consider a range of issues and to protect confidentiality at all cost, and those parameters dictated the kind of case presentation we could offer.

We started with cases with which we were familiar, taking Huntington disease as our paradigm case. We then moved to HD cases that arose from the experience of clinics with which we did not have immediate contact, finally enlarging our focus to include disorders that share with HD an autosomal dominant pattern of inheritance. We had several reasons for proceeding in this way. To begin with, we assume that it is helpful to know what one is talking about. Our group includes extensive experience in HD counseling, and we had easy access to other relevant clinical and scientific expertise bearing on HD. Furthermore, presymptomatic genetic counseling has been most intensively studied in the context of HD; we can expect the move from research, to identification of markers, to linkage testing, to gene identification and direct testing to be followed for other genetic disorders.

As a practical matter, it was difficult to obtain cases to analyze from beyond our own experience. Some of the persons with whom we corresponded had interesting and significant cases to report, but they had not been recorded in a form that could be shared; others preferred to reserve their cases for analyses they planned to conduct themselves. Eventually, we collected additional cases on HD as well as cases involving testing for autosomal dominant polycystic kidney disease (ADPKD), familial adenomatous polyposis (FAP), and familial breast cancer. As is the case with HD, problems associated with recessive inheritance are not at issue for those disorders; however, they present morally relevant differences in penetrance, prognosis, and pathology.

Our sample of cases primarily features HD, with six cases concerning other autosomal dominant diseases. We mean to be clear that our work applies only to a limited sample of genetic diseases, but we think it is a particularly important sample. The history of research on HD and briefer descriptions of research on the other disorders appear in the next section.

We did not begin with a principled choice of which issue to take on first; instead, we began with cases that we believed (often mistakenly) to be simple. In reasoning about individual cases, we began by trying to get as clear as we could about the biological, medical, social, and legal facts. We tried to understand the perspectives of the players in each case: consultands, counselors, family members, and others. We then asked ourselves what moral issues seemed to be raised in this situation and which of the moral considerations seemed to be trump. Readers who can find a consistent utilitarian, deontological, or other moral theory behind the moral considerations we advance will have surpassed the authors of the study. We neither boast of nor apologize for this fact. (Indeed, we are not agreed on the possibility or importance of a comprehensive form of ethical theory.) The persuasiveness of what we have to say about each case must stand on its own merits.

At any rate, moral reasoning as we have attempted it is not readily distinguishable from clear thinking about any kind of problem, moral or otherwise. Our approach is "casuistical" in being case based and related to an emerging professional tradition—that of genetic counseling. Moreover, we make heavy use of precedent and analogy; insofar as possible, we try to resolve one case with reference to our conclusions about others. But we are more eclectic in our use of analytical tools and distinctions than a rigorous casuist might be. (See Jonsen and Toulmin 1988 and Miller 1996.)

Although our method of attack was arbitrary, we have *presented* our cases in a somewhat structured order. We begin with cases in which the testing of one individual will yield information a family member does not want to know; one recurring issue is whether the choice not to learn one's genetic status should prevent someone else from learning that information about him- or herself. Next we move to issues arising when persons do not want information about themselves—or do not want others to know of their risk. That leads us to consider a series of cases in which dangers or benefits to others from testing decisions are at issue. In conclusion, we discuss the testing of children and other consultands for whom testing may be inappropriate or whose ability to consent to testing may be compromised. There is nothing sacred about our organization of these materials, nor are the complexities of the cases captured in this classification. To a significant degree, the analyses are a seamless web that can be entered at any point and will draw the reader in multiple directions.

It was tempting to stop at the level of case analysis, but we felt we should go beyond that and attempt to generalize from our findings. Thus we offer some generalizations in our "Guidelines and Commentary." The Guidelines are topically focused; in them we attempt to identify themes that come up again and again. They include the role of genetic counselors, the significance of ethics in genetic counseling, the importance of counseling, the status of testing protocols, the importance of confidentiality, the legitimacy of the exercise of professional judgment, the right of consultands not to learn their genetic status, and the priority of the consultand's interests. We stress the importance of informed consent, resist attempts to force reproductive choices on parents, and offer a discriminating judgment on the testing of children.

These issues have come up repeatedly in the cases, and we have felt obligated to take a stand on them. So it is possible to use our book in reverse order, starting with the Guidelines and allowing the case references they contain to lead to specific cases. We hope the book will be useful when approached in this more topical way, but we believe that a thoughtful reader will quickly see the extent to which the discussions are intertwined and will recognize that the Guidelines are rooted in the case analyses.

Huntington Disease

We began our three-year project by focusing on Huntington disease, the most studied of a significant class of late-onset, autosomal dominant diseases. Over the past decade, presymptomatic testing for HD has progressed through a full cycle of developmental stages from identification of genetic markers through development of direct gene testing. This history of evolving diagnostic capabilities is likely to be repeated as the mutations for other disorders are mapped and sequenced. Experience with HD has provided a model, guiding much of the thinking about presymptomatic testing for other late-onset genetic diseases, such as breast cancer and Alzheimer disease, which may replicate that developmental cycle within a matter of months. As the pace of research has accelerated, the opportunity to amass information during each stage for each disease may be gone forever. As a result, the lessons learned from the example of HD may provide our only guide as we attempt to cope with the explosion of genetic knowledge.

A brief history of the HD experience will illustrate the path likely to be followed as other late-onset genetic diseases are mapped and sequenced through efforts supported by the Human Genome Project.

Huntington disease is the most common inherited neurological disorder, with a prevalence ranging from 4.1 to 7.5 cases per 100,000 in Caucasians (Folstein 1989). HD is inherited in an autosomal dominant pattern; each child of a parent affected with the disorder has a 50 percent chance of inheriting the HD mutation. Penetrance of HD is close to 100 percent, and most people who inherit the mutation begin to show the classic symptoms of the disease in their late thirties or early forties. However, the disease has been found to occur as young as two years of age and as old as seventy (Hayden 1981). An estimated 3 percent to 10 percent of cases present with symptom onset prior to the age of twenty and about 90 percent of so-called juvenile cases of HD are inherited from the father (Harper 1991). The symptoms of HD include abnormal involuntary movements (chorea) accompanied by intellectual impairment (dementia) and a variety of psychiatric disturbances, most commonly depression (Conneally 1984). Death normally occurs ten to seventeen years after onset (Harper 1991).

HD has been characterized as a disease of the basal ganglia, which are involved in cognitive and emotional disorders as well as impairment of motor functioning (Folstein 1989). Although some medications have been helpful in treating the characteristic movements of HD and psychiatric symptoms, no treatment is available for the underlying disorder, and no cure has been found.

Mapping the Gene

In 1983, Huntington disease became the first disease to be mapped to a previously unknown location through the use of restriction enzymes, which cleave deoxyrybonucleic acid (DNA) at sequence-specific sites (Gusella et al. 1983). Inherited variations of these DNA sequences, also known as restriction fragment length polymorphisms or RFLPs, can be used as genetic markers to map diseases on chromosomes as well as to trace the inheritance of diseases within families. Subsequent studies confirmed and refined the gene's association with the initial marker on the short arm of chromosome 4 (Folstein et al. 1985; Conneally et al. 1989), and the identification of various additional markers soon followed (Wasmuth et al. 1988; Whaley et al. 1988; Youngman et al. 1988). The discovery of polymorphic markers linked to HD was a significant advance in HD research. Not only did it provide a possible clue for finding the gene and to understanding the mechanism for how the gene caused brain cells to die, the discovery also meant that predictive testing for those at risk for HD was possible.

The presymptomatic test procedure, called a linkage test, compares the marker DNA of family members affected with HD with the DNA of unaffected family members who were at risk for HD, but who have outlived the age of onset in their family and are old enough to have only a very slight chance of developing HD. These elderly relatives are called "escapees."

Predictive testing using linkage has several drawbacks. First, blood or tissue samples are needed from several family members, both affected and elderly unaffected relatives. The exact family members from whom samples are needed varies for each family and must be determined on a case-by-case basis. Estimates were that only 15 percent (Harper and Sarafazi 1985) to 37 percent (Misra et al. 1988) of families with HD would have the requisite structure or samples available to allow testing using linkage. In families that did have the necessary structure, gathering the needed samples was often time-consuming, required delicate negotiations with estranged relatives, and effectively precluded confidentiality for the person being tested, at least within the family.

Second, accurate information regarding the status of all individuals donating samples is crucial, whether or not they are affected with HD. Neurological examinations and/or medical records had to be obtained for each person. Family members thus ran the risk that their relatives would learn something about their medical history or their current neurological status that they might not have sought on their own and with which they might not be ready to cope.

Third, testing using linkage is not 100 percent accurate. Estimates of the error rate of linkage testing are based on the distance between the gene itself and the markers used for testing. Early tests were estimated as about 90 percent to 95 percent accurate. With the discovery of markers more closely linked to the HD gene, accuracy increased to 99 percent in a fairly short time.

Fourth, linkage testing was expensive. Commercial laboratories offering testing charged approximately $500 per sample, and the average test required four to five samples. Testing was also labor-intensive; each case involved long hours of analyzing pedigrees, collecting the necessary samples, and gathering and reviewing medical records. Even so, test results might still be uninformative.

Predictive Testing

In preparation for predictive testing for HD, a workshop on pre-symptomatic diagnosis was convened in 1985 by Dr. Milton Wexler, President of the Hereditary Disease Foundation and the father of two daughters at risk for HD. Invited participants were laypersons with an interest in HD, as well as researchers and clinicians with years of experience in working closely with HD patients and their families. The group concluded that testing should be introduced on an experimental basis and that release of genetic probes for more widespread testing should await the findings of these experimental programs. Other members of the genetics community attacked this approach as extremely paternalistic.

The workshop also developed preliminary guidelines for predictive testing protocols, including eligibility criteria and screening procedures. These protocols included a neurological examination, psychiatric screening, intensive pretest counseling and posttest follow-up. The experimental protocols were designed to determine (1) the psychiatric, psychological, and social consequences of informing people of their genetic status with regard to HD; (2) whether pretest characteristics could distinguish those who adapt well to knowledge of their genetic status from those who adapt poorly; and (3) whether educational and therapeutic interventions could mitigate morbid psychological and social outcomes (Brandt et al. 1989).

In September 1986, centers at Massachusetts General Hospital in Boston and the Johns Hopkins Hospital in Baltimore began offering pre-symptomatic testing for HD on an experimental basis. Other centers offering testing using similar protocols opened in Canada (Bloch et al. 1989; Fox et al. 1989), Wales (Morris et al. 1989), England (Craufurd et al. 1989), Belgium (Evers-Kiebooms 1990), the Netherlands (Tibben et al. 1990) and Australia (Turner et al. 1988).

The Development of Guidelines for Testing

In 1989 the Huntington's Disease Society of America (HDSA) published *Guidelines for Predictive Testing for Huntington's Disease*. These guidelines reflected the cooperative efforts of scientists, doctors, health professionals, HD patients and their families, and those who were offering testing. Prominent features included mandatory counseling, the assumption of informed choice on the part of the test taker including criteria for those deemed unable to make an informed choice, and restriction of the test to those aged eighteen or older except when a pregnancy was involved.

In 1985 a committee of representatives of the International Huntington Association (IHA) and the World Federation of Neurology (WFN) Research Group on Huntington's Chorea was established specifically to produce recommendations for the use of the predictive test for HD. At their respective meetings in Vancouver in 1989, the two organizations reviewed and adopted these recommendations.

Although similar in spirit, the HDSA and IHA-WFN guidelines differ in format and content. The HDSA guidelines presented a model protocol to be used for testing, describing in detail the number, content, and length of counseling sessions. In contrast, the IHA-WFN guidelines ("Ethical Issues Policy Statement on Huntington's Disease Molecular Genetics Predictive Test") presented a series of recommendations and commentary. The IHA-WFN product is both broader in scope and more specific in delineating exactly how testing should be used.

In most cases, our guidelines agree with the recommendations of the HDSA and the IHA-WFN, both of which were revised when the gene for HD was found in 1993. Specifically, we agree on the need for a team approach, the importance of counseling, the fact that testing may be postponed or denied in limited circumstances, and a presumption against testing children.

Some areas of disagreement are evident, however. The 1989 HDSA guidelines strongly recommend against so-called secret testing, which is discussed here in Case 23, "Emily," and suggest a minimum number of counseling sessions, an issue addressed in Case 24, "Mrs. K." In contrast, we would authorize this kind of testing and would object to a minimum number of counseling sessions.

The 1990 IHA-WFN guidelines state, "Tests should not be performed that provide diagnostic information about another person who has not requested the test except in unique circumstances." We disagree. We address this issue in Cases 1, "Paul and Michael"; 2, "Father and Son"; and 6, "Kirsten and David."

In the revised (1994) IHA-WFN guidelines, a majority of representatives to the International Huntington Association asked that an additional comment be added to this debate as follows: "If there is a conflicting situation in a family, when a young individual wants to be tested but his/her parent at risk does not want to know their status, the right of the adult child should have priority over the right of the parent not to know." Ultimately, the group reached a compromise. Recommendation 2.4 was changed to read, "Extreme care should be exercised when testing would provide information about another person who has not requested the test." The commentary was expanded to include the following statement: "A considerable majority of representatives from the lay organizations (IHA) feel that if no consensus can be reached, the right of the adult child to know should have priority over the right of the parent not to know." This change considerably narrows the scope of this recommendation and leaves little guidance for the situations found in Cases 1 and 2.

One topic that has prompted intensive discussion in the literature is nondirective counseling. The HDSA and IHA-WFN guidelines do not refer specifically to the issue of nondirectiveness; they offer general statements (e.g., "The decision to take the test is solely the choice of the individual concerned" [IHA-WFN 1994]). This issue seems to us to call for a somewhat more nuanced discussion. On the one hand, we reject the traditional model of nondirective counseling, in which counselors are limited to the value-neutral presentation of information. Rather, we attempt to distinguish among kinds of advice that might be offered. In several of our cases, for example, we urge counselors to press consultands on issues of disclosure. (See Cases 7, "Robert"; 8, "Mr. H."; 9, "Natalie"; 10, "Mary Ann"; and 11, "Maurice." In addition, see Guidelines ID4a, IIA, VB2, VC, and VIIIB.) On the other hand, we identify kinds of value judgments counselors ought not share. Finally, we defend the importance of *professional* values.

The Data

Preliminary findings from the presymptomatic testing projects in Boston and Baltimore soon began to appear in the literature (Brandt et al. 1989; Meissen et al. 1988; Quaid et al. 1987). The results suggested that presymptomatic testing for HD could be safely conducted in a supportive setting with appropriate long-term monitoring of those tested. Subsequent studies offered further support for that conclusion (Bloch et al. 1992; Nance et al. 1991). In light of these findings, additional centers began to offer testing on a clinical basis. By the end of 1991, twenty-three centers were offering presymptomatic testing for HD as a clinical service (Quaid 1993).

Experience has yielded a wealth of information regarding the consequences of predictive testing. Psychological outcome data from the Canadian Collaborative Group has demonstrated the pros and cons of testing for those found to be at increased risk (Bloch et al. 1992) and decreased risk (Huggins et al. 1992). One-year follow-up data on 130 persons tested (including 37 with an increased risk) suggested decreased anxiety and overall improvement in the quality of life of those tested (Wiggins et al. 1992). Six-month follow-up data from the Dutch testing program showed few serious negative outcomes and some improvement in the quality of life of participants (Tibben et al. 1992). Investigators from Johns Hopkins concluded that, although testing appeared to have negative as well as positive consequences regardless of test outcome, the benefits of testing appeared to outweigh the drawbacks (Codori and Brandt 1994). It is important to note, however, that all of these programs followed approved testing protocols including neurological examinations, psychological screening, several sessions of pretest counseling, and posttest follow-up.

The Discovery of the HD Gene

In March 1993, the long-awaited announcement finally came: Researchers had found the gene for HD (Huntington's Disease Collaborative Research Group 1993). The HD gene, called IT15, is an expanded and unstable DNA segment in the Huntington disease gene on chromosome 4p16.3. The expansion is due to the presence of a repeated trinucleotide (CAG_n). The repeating CAG segment is longer on the HD chromosome than on the normal chromosome, which was described by Andrew et al. (1993) as having ten to twenty-nine repeats. Further, the segment is unstable, apparently changing in length during gamete formation. Thus, children may have a larger number of CAG repeats than their parents (Duyao et al. 1993; Snell et al. 1993; Andrew et al. 1993). Recent research suggests that these characteristics of the gene may account for variations in the age of onset and may explain "sporadic" cases of HD, in which an individual develops symptoms in the absence of a family history of the disorder (Gusella and MacDonald 1994).

In individuals with HD, the number of CAG repeats is usually forty or above. Individuals who do not have the HD mutation usually have twenty-six or fewer repeats. Variations in CAG repeat number also appear to include a so-called gray zone variously defined as twenty-seven to thirty-nine (McGlennan et al. 1995), thirty to thirty-eight (Norremolle et al. 1993), thirty-three to thirty-eight (MacMillan and Quinn 1993), and twenty-seven to thirty-nine (American College of Medical Genetics/ American Society of Human Genetics Huntington Disease Genetic Testing Working Group 1998). A recent study reported that no cases of HD have been reported with thirty-five or fewer repeats and that the smallest CAG repeat associated with symptoms of HD is thirty-six. In addition, several elderly individuals with thirty-six to thirty-nine CAG repeats did not appear to have symptoms of HD, suggesting that the HD mutation may not be fully penetrant within this range (Rubinsztein et al. 1996).

Kremer et al. studied 1,007 patients who had received a diagnosis of HD, 113 control subjects with a family history of neurological disorders other than HD, and 1,595 control chromosomes. Of the 1,007 HD patients, they found that 995 patients had CAG repeats ranging from 36 to 121 (with a median of 44). Of the 12 persons whose chromosomes had a smaller number of CAG repeats, 11 showed features atypical of HD on review of clinical records as well as findings from neuropathological examination and positron emission tomography. This group found "intermediate" alleles (which they defined as alleles with 30 to 35 CAG repeats) in 12 of the 1,595 control chromosomes. One fifty-seven-year-old individual was found to have 39 repeats on one chromosome, although she had no symptoms of HD and no family history of the disorder for three generations (Kremer et al. 1994).

The range of CAG_n corresponding to the foregoing categories (high probability of HD, indeterminate, low probability of HD) has not been unequivocally established. However, based on the most recent research findings, the suggested categories are as follows:

26 and below = normal
27–35 repeats = nonpenetrant with meiotic instability
36–39 repeats = variably penetrant with meiotic instability
40 and above = HD (American College of Medical Genetics/American Society of Human Genetics Huntington Disease Genetic Testing Working Group 1998).

Direct Testing

Direct testing for the HD mutation through the use of polymerase chain reaction (PCR) has greatly simplified the technical aspects of genetic testing for HD. It is now possible to test an individual without samples from other family members, although many centers recommend that at least one closely related affected individual be tested in order to confirm the HD mutation in the family. This recommendation is intended to ensure that the disorder in the family is correctly diagnosed as HD by confirmation of an expanded CAG repeat. Following this recommendation has enabled many centers to identify families previously thought to have HD who do not have the HD mutation.

Testing for HD is now faster, simpler, more accurate, more affordable, and more widely available. These technical advances and economic improvements have not changed the emotional impact of test results, however. In fact, they have raised concerns that are now coming to fruition. Freed from the need to take extensive family histories and gather blood samples and medical records from several family members, more centers are offering testing and more professionals are ordering these tests, many of whom have had little experience with HD or predictive genetic testing. Individuals are being tested with little prior preparation, little counseling, and sometimes questionable information pertaining to the interpretation of test results or the natural history of HD. Freed from the strict requirements of research protocols designed to collect data about the consequences of testing, individuals who choose to be tested more closely reflect the general population at risk for HD. Some evidence suggests that these individuals may be less psychologically adjusted and have less support than those tested early on using generally accepted standards of testing (Adam et al. 1995). Consequently, testing for these individuals may pose a higher risk of negative outcomes.

Other Disorders of Interest

In addition to HD, our cases feature three other autosomal dominant, late-onset genetic diseases. Because these disorders differ in significant ways from HD, genetic counseling and testing raise new issues. Here we outline the salient characteristics of the disorders featured in our cases.

Familial Adenomatous Polyposis

Familial adenomatous polyposis (FAP) affects the gastrointestinal tract. The condition is also known as hereditary polyposis of the colon, familial polyposis, and Gardner syndrome. The incidence of FAP has been estimated to be approximately 1 in 8,000 to 1 in 10,000 (Petersen 1994). Typically, an individual with FAP will develop hundreds of polyps throughout the entire gastrointestinal system but primarily in the colon. The major risk associated with this condition is cancer, which inevitably arises from the polyps (Bulow 1987). The adenomatous polyposis coli (APC) gene, located on chromosome 5 at band q21 (Nishisho et al. 1991), is responsible for FAP. A germline mutation of the APC gene is transmitted as an autosomal dominant trait. Because the gene is a tumor suppressor gene, both copies of the gene must be inactivated in neoplasia (Powell, Petersen et al. 1992). In other words, individuals with a germline mutation of a tumor suppressor gene need a "knockout" or second acquired mutation of the second (normal) allele for cancer to develop in a specific tissue. In effect, a germline mutation of a tumor suppressor gene is transmitted as an autosomal dominant trait, but the development of cancer can be considered recessive at the cellular level.

Because onset of FAP can occur in childhood, screening for the presence of polyps is recommended to begin around age eleven (Petersen et al. 1991). In contrast to Huntington disease, the disease course of FAP may be modified by surgical procedures including colectomy and resection of desmoid tumors. The fact that most of the FAP mutations produce an aberrant protein enabled the development of a protein truncation test in 1993 (Powell, Petersen et al. 1992). This test is used for genetic testing in both symptomatic and asymptomatic individuals.

Genetic testing for FAP raises issues that differ from those related to testing for Huntington disease. FAP typically has an earlier onset, but, more importantly, medical intervention is available that can reduce morbidity and mortality. We have included FAP cases for the very purpose of challenging decisions made in the context of HD. For example, we reach quite different conclusions with regard to genetic testing of children for FAP. (See Case 16, "Harriet.")

Autosomal Dominant Polycystic Kidney Disease

Another inherited syndrome featured in our cases and commentary is autosomal dominant polycystic kidney disease. ADPKD is a common disorder with a prevalence of approximately 1/1,000 (Davies et al. 1991). As the name implies, this disorder is characterized by cyst formation in multiple organs, primarily the kidney, but also the genitourinary and gastrointestinal systems. Complications of the syndrome include hypertension, end-stage renal disease (ESRD), cardiac abnormalities, and intracranial aneurysms. (Gabow 1993) Apparently, the cysts increase in number and size over time, destroying the normal architecture of the tissue (Grantham 1995). Age of onset of cysts is variable and can occur anytime during one's life. End-stage renal disease typically develops in late middle age, with average onset at 55 years (Bear 1995). Renal transplantation is the treatment of choice once renal failure occurs (Hannig et al. 1991).

ADPKD is genetically heterogeneous; to date, two loci have been identified. One gene (PKD1) is located on the short arm of chromosome 16 (Reeders et al. 1985); the other (PKD2) is on the long arm of chromosome 4 (Kimberling et al. 1993). Mutations of PKD1 are thought to account for 85 percent to 90 percent of ADPKD cases (Peike et al. 1989).

Ultrasound imaging of the kidneys is used to detect renal cysts in presymptomatic individuals. However, it is estimated that the probability of detecting an asymptomatic ADPKD heterozygote with renal ultrasound is estimated to be only 86 percent by age twenty-five. The probability of a false negative diagnosis in individuals over age 30 has been estimated to be equal to or less than 13 percent (Bear et al. 1984). Linkage analysis has been used to determine gene status in unaffected and presymptomatic individuals. Now that PKD1 has been cloned (International Polycystic Kidney Disease Consortium 1995; Hughes et al. 1995), direct gene testing will become available.

Discussion of testing in this genetic disorder must take into consideration the special circumstance that gene-negative family members may be pressured to donate a healthy kidney to an affected relative.

Familial Breast Cancer

Finally, two of our cases involve genetic testing for breast cancer. Like ADPKD, breast cancer is common. It is the leading cause of cancer in women. In 1996 the American Cancer Society estimated that approximately 185,000 American women would develop breast cancer and 44,500 women would die from breast cancer that year (Parker et al. 1996). The lifetime risk of developing breast cancer for women in the general population is 1 in 8 (American Cancer Society 1995). However, some women have a much higher lifetime risk of developing breast and/ or ovarian cancer than that of the general population. Inherited susceptibility becomes apparent through occurrence of the same (or related) neoplasm in several members of a family, earlier age at presentation, multifocality in the affected organ, and bilaterality of disease in paired organs. Hereditary breast cancer syndromes identified to date include the Li Fraumeni syndrome, Cowden's syndrome, site-specific breast cancer, and familial breast and ovarian cancer. It is estimated that hereditary breast cancer accounts for 5 percent to 10 percent of all breast cancer cases.

In 1990, Mary Claire King's group announced linkage in families with early-onset breast cancer to a region localized on the long arm of chromosome 17 (Hall et al. 1990). In October 1994, a collaborative group led by Mark Skolnick identified the DNA sequence of this gene, BRCA1 (Miki et al. 1994). Another breast cancer gene, BRCA2, was mapped to the long arm of chromosome 13 and subsequently cloned in 1995 (Wooster et al. 1995). Both are thought to be tumor-suppressor genes (Miki et al. 1994). A woman with an inherited mutation of either gene has a risk of approximately 85 percent of developing breast cancer during her lifetime (Easton et al. 1995; Ford et al. 1994). Gene mutations of BRCA1 also increase the risk for ovarian cancer, elevating the lifetime risk to 45 percent to 60 percent and increasing risks of colon cancer and prostate cancer in men (Easton et al. 1995; Ford et al. 1994). Onset of disease in gene carriers is generally earlier than that observed for the general population, often occurring before menopause but rarely in adolescence (FitzGerald et al. 1996; Langston et al. 1996).

Approximately 100 gene mutations of the BRCA1 gene have been identified and are found scattered throughout this very large gene (Collins 1996). New mutations must be interpreted cautiously, to be certain that they are associated with disease and are not rare polymorphisms or clinically insignificant variants. As a result, testing for BRCA1 mutations has proceeded slowly, as research laboratories continue to gather and interpret information regarding mutations in individual families.

For women with inherited mutations of BRCA1 or BRCA2, recommended screening modalities include breast self-examination, examination by a physician, and mammography. However, despite diligent screening, disease may develop, and outcome may not be improved. Prophylactic mastectomy or oophorectomy may considerably lower the risk for the development of cancer, but will not eliminate it.

Breast cancer is another disorder for which medical or surgical intervention may modify the disease course. Case 5, "Carol," addresses whether a surgeon should perform prophylactic surgery without knowledge of the patient's BRCA1 test results. Case 10, "Mary Anne," asks whether a health care provider should override a request for confidentiality when a daughter's positive BRCA1 test result reveals that her mother's risk is elevated beyond the risk estimated from family history. Genetic counselors and medical practitioners alike will certainly find themselves in the center of situations such as these.

Cases

Case 1 *Paul and Michael*

Paul, a healthy twenty-five-year-old man, contacts a testing center to request genetic testing for Huntington disease. Paul's father has HD. The father and his family live in another part of the country and are not known to the center. Paul has an identical twin brother, Michael, who does not wish to have the predictive test.

Paul has moved away from his family for work reasons, but he maintains regular telephone contact with his parents, twin brother, and older sister. Paul is planning to get married; he and his partner, Linda, are determined to find out whether he will develop HD before they start a family. Michael is single and, according to Paul, does not think he could cope with the knowledge if he knew that he carried the HD mutation.

Paul understands that his test result will reveal Michael's gene status. He states that he will not tell Michael or other family members that he is undergoing the predictive test. If he receives a positive result, he says that he will not tell Michael. However, he might tell Michael if he were to receive a negative result.

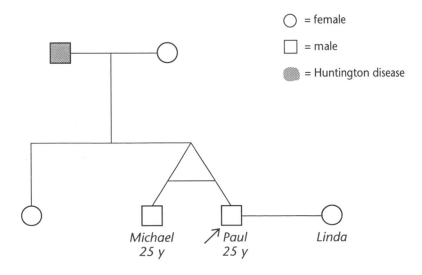

○ = female

□ = male

● = Huntington disease

Michael
25 y

Paul
25 y

Linda

This case raises difficult ethical questions for both the counselor and the patient; our focus is on the counselor, but the patient must be treated as a moral agent in his own right.

The first issue is whether the counselor should authorize testing for Paul. It is convenient to resolve this question by focusing on the interests of the concerned parties. Paul, Michael, Linda, their potential offspring, and society may have interests that deserve consideration.

Paul has the full range of autonomy interests normally associated with reproductive decision making and awareness of one's own medical condition. He is in a patient-professional relationship with the counselor and may expect her to give his interests primary concern. Although neither Linda nor Michael is the counselor's consultand, both have relevant interests. Linda has an interest in knowing the genetic health of the man she plans to marry and in being able to make informed reproductive decisions; Michael has an interest in not having unwanted personal information forced upon him and an interest in not being thrust into a situation with which he cannot cope. His interest is taken very seriously by the Huntington's Disease Society of America. HDSA's guidelines specifically address the situation in which individuals seek testing while their at-risk parents are still living:

> The potential impact on other family members needs to be considered. For some parents, the prospect of this information is not particularly anxiety-provoking. For other parents in other families, however, the impact of this information may be substantial. Professionals offering this type of testing should explore the family dynamics and try to assess the implications for other family members. A consensus on testing among those individuals who are directly affected is the ideal situation, although this will not always be possible. (HDSA 1994, 12)

The case presents two other interests of possible relevance, but we reject consideration of either. First, some may argue that Paul and Linda's unconceived children have interests to consider. But if unconceived children have interests, it is hard to know whether they have an interest in having a life, or in avoiding the suffering of HD or being at risk for HD. Because it is unclear whether the unconceived have interests and because reasoning about those interests—if any—is therefore so speculative, they should be treated as irrelevant to the resolution of this dilemma.

Second, some may argue that society has an interest in preventing the births of persons at risk for HD. However, consideration of this aggregated social interest is problematic on moral grounds. In general, if a counselor considers society's interests, those interests will almost surely prevail, to the detriment of individuals to whom the counselor owes a fiduciary obligation. Serious consideration of an overall social interest opens the door to eugenic and cost-saving decisions. Further ethical analysis becomes moot, and the interests of identifiable human beings are overridden. The danger of such an approach is apparent. Therefore, society's interests should be treated as irrelevant for the purpose of deciding whether the counselor should authorize testing for Paul.

Paul's and Linda's reasons for wanting the test are important, not just idle curiosity. They seek testing before marriage and prior to reproducing. If Paul is found not to carry the HD mutation, then there is no risk that any children that he might have will carry the mutation.

One option that might be considered is nondisclosing prenatal testing using linkage. Using this procedure, it would be possible to determine whether a fetus was at the same level of risk as Paul or at very low risk. (See the Glossary for an explanation of nondisclosing prenatal testing.) The point of using this procedure is that Paul and Linda would be able to determine whether any given pregnancy had an approximately 50 percent risk for HD or a very low risk. Paul's genetic status would not be revealed, and, therefore, neither would Michael's.

However, this procedure has several drawbacks. First, Linda would actually have to become pregnant. In nondisclosing prenatal testing, linkage analysis would be used. Blood samples for analysis would be needed from Paul's parents, Paul, and Linda. Second, a fetal sample would be taken either by chorionic villus sampling or amniocentesis, thus subjecting Linda to discomfort as well as the risk of miscarriage or fetal malformation (Rhoads et al. 1989; Crandall et al. 1994). If the results of the linkage analysis indicate that the fetus is at the same level of risk as Paul, Paul and Linda face a dilemma. They must either terminate a pregnancy at 50 percent risk, or they must continue the pregnancy with the knowledge that if Paul begins to show symptoms, that will mean that their child carries the HD mutation and will develop the disorder as well.

The psychological burden on Linda and Paul of possible fetal exclusion testing is at least as serious as the threat to Michael's psychic well-being posed by direct presymptomatic testing of Paul. Moreover, increasing the possibility of either terminating a pregnancy or potentially learning that a child carries the HD mutation, adds another, unnecessary, dimension of potential tragedy to this case.[1]

On balance, Paul's interests, augmented by Linda's interests, outweigh Michael's interests. The issue is clearer if stated in the following

---

1. Of course, testing now does not guarantee that the issue of prenatal testing will never arise. If Paul's test is positive and he and Linda decide to reproduce, the issue of prenatal testing may confront them at that time.

terms: How can one withhold important health information from someone—information that will affect marriage and reproduction—because
the information *may* (depending on the result of the test and the circumstances of the untested twin) be devastating to his brother? How could
we conclude that Michael's choice not to learn his risk rightly forces the
same choice, possible abortion, the sacrifice of parenthood, or the knowing creation of children at risk for a serious disease onto Paul and Linda?

If the facts of this case differed in certain ways, it would be harder
to resolve. Specifically, if both Michael and Paul were the counselor's patients, or if Michael were under psychiatric care, the resolution would be
more complicated.

If both Michael and Paul were the counselor's patients, then the
counselor would clearly owe obligations to each of them. If Michael were
also a consultand, one serious problem presented by this case would
be different. As it stands, we have only Paul's *report* on Michael's situation. Paul may misunderstand or seriously underestimate his brother. If
Michael were also a consultand, the counselor could assess Michael's
situation for herself.

On the other hand, with two consultands in the same family, a
counselor must deal with situations in which their interests conflict.
When patients' interests are as closely intertwined as they are in this
case, mechanical approaches (e.g., saying the counselor's primary obligation is to Paul when she is dealing with him and to Michael when she is
dealing with Michael) will not work.

Conceding her duty to both men, the counselor should first try to
resolve the conflict between their interests. If that fails, she should try to
balance their interests. She can reduce the conflict of interest between
Michael and Paul to some degree by counseling Paul directively about
the importance of keeping information from Michael and trying to get
Paul to agree to do so. It would be naive, however, to rely on such a
promise. Balancing the twins' competing interests is best approximated
through disclosure to Paul combined with discussion of his responsibilities.

We would need more facts to appreciate the full significance of
Michael's being "under psychiatric care." Importantly, being under psychiatric care may suggest not only increased risk but increased professional assistance. If Michael is receiving professional help, that support
might mitigate any negative consequences of learning his brother's test
results. Risk to Michael is relevant, but in our view it is most relevant to
Paul's obligations, to which we now turn.

Suppose Paul is tested. We think the counselor has an obligation to
discuss Paul's responsibilities with him. He and Linda want the diagnos-

tic information "before starting a family." What actions do they contemplate if a test is positive? Will they not have children if Paul carries the HD mutation, or will they opt for prenatal testing and engage in selective abortion, or will they reproduce with full knowledge of the risk they are running? The counselor should attempt to determine their intentions and should counsel with awareness of the gravity of their options. While coercion, such as extracting a promise not to reproduce as a condition of testing, would be inefficacious and arguably unethical (see Case 18, "Mr. and Mrs. B."), the full range of options, together with their risks and benefits should be explored with the couple. Neutral, flatly presented "nondirective" information places the consultand's decision in a vacuum and ignores what the counselor knows about the suffering associated with HD, the social reaction to abortion, and its possible psychological effects on Linda and Paul.

In addition, testing Paul has risks for his brother. Michael should not be asked to run those risks unless Paul intends to do more than satisfy his curiosity. The counselor should offer the test after the options have been explored, but in our opinion Paul—out of regard for Michael—should not be tested unless either Michael changes his mind or the reasons for testing are serious. In this case they are serious, and they relate to Paul and Linda's plans to have a family, but they key on a decision not to have children carrying the HD mutation. That decision can be effectuated in several ways: Paul and Linda can avoid conception and adopt; they can use artificial insemination by donor, preimplantation diagnosis, or other sophisticated technologies for reproduction; or Linda can be impregnated by Paul, undergo prenatal testing, and abort any fetuses who carry the HD mutation. All of these options raise ethical issues. The justification for Paul's decision to be tested relates to his and Linda's willingness to use one or more of these options, if he tests positive.

Moreover, Paul's obligation to avoid harming his brother clearly requires him to refrain from telling anyone beyond the absolutely necessary circle of persons who must be informed that he is seeking testing and from reporting the test results. The solace Paul might receive from discussing his status with his family cannot justify hurting another person, especially a close relative.

In conclusion, we believe that on the facts as presented, Paul should be offered the HD test, but it is part of the counselor's responsibility to counsel him about the complexity of his options. (See Heimler and Zanko 1995.)

Case 2 *Father and Son*

Mr. K. is forty-four years old and has a 50 percent risk for HD. He has had several episodes of clinical depression in the past and has not pursued predictive testing because he is not sure that he would be able to handle the information. Mr. K. has a twenty-four-year-old son who is thinking of getting married. Now that direct gene testing is possible, Mr. K's son has approached the testing center about being tested. He considers it his right to obtain this information, and, although he is aware of the potential ramifications for his father, he wishes to pursue testing.

Like Case 1, "Paul and Michael," this case raises the central issue of testing one individual when another family member about whom the test may be informative has chosen not to discover his risk of carrying the HD gene. In both cases, one person's self-image will be jeopardized if another family member gains information about himself. This case differs in that it presents the situation of parent and child, not siblings.

The responsibilities and rights of parents and children may well be distinguishable from those of siblings. Indeed, our analysis of cases involving the testing of children depends on a view of special parental rights and duties (see Cases 13, "Mr. Crawford"; 14, "Mr. and Mrs. Anderson"; 15, "Jimmy"; 16, "Harriet"; and 17, "Charley"). Parents are expected to assume primary responsibilities for care during a child's formative years; some level of renunciation of parental self-interest is expected when children are growing up. Later in life, grown children may be expected to assume responsibility for ill or aging parents. These relationships, as well as relationships among siblings, may have all shades of emotional color, ranging from close bonds of love to estrangement, alienation, indifference, or hate. It does not require much imagination to fill in details in this case so as to make the son's request for testing cold and heartless—or, in stark contrast, a praiseworthy acceptance of responsibility.

In thinking about this case, we imagined a hypothetical scenario, one in which a forty-year-old man at risk for HD contemplates remarriage and having a second family. He wants to be tested before marriage. His seventeen-year-old son, however, has no wish to learn more about his genetic status. In what ways would our verdict in this hypothetical case differ from our judgment about the present case? We were forced to the conclusion that both cases present decisive issues bearing on intimacy and personal stability rather than on the morally asymmetrical character of the relationship between parents and children.

Thus, we see no reason to decide this case differently from Case 1, "Paul and Michael." One family member's preferences, even justified choices, are not in themselves a sufficient reason to refuse a test to another family member. The scenario would have differed in the era of linkage studies, when the father would have had to be involved in the process from the beginning. In linkage testing, the father could impede, perhaps veto, his son's quest for knowledge by refusing to give a blood sample; that would lead to an important question of whether he *ought* to do so. With the availability of direct gene testing, however, he can be completely bypassed.

We conclude that the son has a right to information that will allow him to ignore his father's wishes. The fact and the character of a relationship are of great relevance, but we cannot generalize about the claims made by parents, children, siblings, or lovers, even in the special case of the relationship between parents and children.

As in Case 1, our decision turns on our conviction that it is appropriate to give persons information they seek about their gene status, information of obvious relevance to fundamental choices they may make. The justification for testing does not rest solely on the immediate likelihood of reproduction. The differences in the formality of the relationship between "partners" and the son and his intended in this case are not decisive—either may involve reproduction; even if we were to try to take the interests of possible children into account, there is obviously no way of telling which of these settings is more likely to serve their putative interests.

As in Case 1, we are aware of the possibility that our conclusion may lead to a destructive result for some concerned parties. As in that case, however, we think it is preferable to counsel the consultand regarding the possible detrimental effects on other family members rather than to refuse testing. To the extent possible, every effort should be made to include other family members about whom information may be learned in counseling so that a satisfactory resolution to the conflict can be obtained.

In both cases of family conflict among adults, we are forced to a permissive conclusion on access to testing, but we balance that with a conviction about the nature of counseling of tested persons. Specifically, we think it is incumbent on genetic counselors to assist consultands pro-actively in thinking through the choices they will be forced to make. This obligation may mean adoption of what John Arras has called a "moral education" model of counseling in which the counselor "would not tell the [consultands] what they think [they] ought to do" but would "attempt to confront" consultands with "the full force of the moral dilemmas" actually at stake (Arras 1990, 374). It might mean "negotiated directive counseling" in which consultands agree to ask the counselor's recommendation—which would have to be given with sensitivity to the consultand's own values (Arras 1990 375f). At a minimum, the counselor must discuss with the son his father's feelings, circumstances, and prospects.

Our ultimate rationale for this view of counseling is our belief that counselors are more than a source of information, as the title *counselor* implies. Here, the counselor should relate to the son as a moral agent, exploring with him the implications of his choices for his father and others. She or he should establish a collaborative relationship in which it is credible to offer him advice, which might include the possibility of keeping the fact of the test from his father or strategies for discussing the results with Mr. K. The right choice for the son to make will be a function of facts much more complex than those presented in this short summary, but in this case he should be tested if he so chooses.

Case 3 Sarah

Sarah sought predictive testing for HD. She expressed concern about possible symptoms of HD as well as considerable anxiety about her children's risk of developing the disorder.

Sarah's psychological evaluation revealed no evidence of illness or instability. When she provided a blood sample for the presymptomatic test, she asked when the results would be available. Center staff explained that the analysis is usually completed within ten days, although it can take longer.

Sarah said that returning in ten days would be impossible. She scheduled a visit to learn tentative results at seventeen days, assuming the procedure would be completed at that time.

On Day 10, the clinic staff learned that Sarah does not carry the HD mutation. The test results are highly accurate.

On Day 11, the staff received a letter from Sarah stating that she has decided not to return for the test result. She wrote that she prefers to live with the hope that the test is negative, rather than having to face the certainty that the test is positive.

Some commentators would have an easy time with this case. Sarah's competence is not in question, and she has chosen not to receive her test results. That decision is her own. Respect for her autonomy might indicate that the counselor should simply leave it at that. While we think the question is harder than this approach suggests, our conclusion is the same.

Unfortunately, complicating factors are apparent, including Sarah's obvious ambivalence just within the past month, as well as the fact that she and the counselor are parties to a fiduciary relationship, which carries some moral responsibilities of beneficence on the part of the counselor. The counselor must think through the question of Sarah's best interests, even if this reflection proves insufficient to resolve the problem. It is tempting for the counselor to push this good news onto Sarah.

Sarah's situation is understandable. The fear of loss of health is normal, and anxiety develops when ill health threatens. In this case, that anxiety centers on disclosure of test results, which may indicate that she carries a gene mutation for Huntington disease, a disease for which there currently is no treatment or cure. Perhaps Sarah has held out hope that she will not be afflicted with HD. Now the judgment day is at hand, and that hope may be destroyed. Recognizing the 50 percent chance of an unfavorable result, Sarah prefers to avoid the judgment; she therefore chooses not to learn her test results.

She is not alone. Analyzing data collected before testing was available, various studies estimated that 56 percent to 77 percent of individuals at risk would request presymptomatic gene testing (Kessler et al. 1987; Mastromauro et al. 1987; Meissen and Bercheck 1987; Markel et al. 1987). When linkage testing became available, the demand was much less than expected; one study found only 9 percent to 15 percent of individuals at risk for HD requesting testing (Quaid 1993). Respondents' reasons for declining presymptomatic testing for HD included: (1) the lack of an effective cure; (2) loss of health insurance; (3) increased risk for children; (4) financial cost of testing; and (5) inability to "undo" the knowledge. Moreover, 25 percent to 30 percent of those who commit to testing change their minds and decide against it (Wiggins et al. 1992, Quaid and Morris 1993).

The effect on participants of learning their risk status is unclear. When protocols for risk-altering testing were established, considerable speculation surrounded the psychological consequences of predictive testing for Huntington disease (Kessler et al. 1987; Hayden et al. 1988; Meissen et al. 1988; Wasmuth et al. 1988; Brandt et al. 1989). Data are now emerging on the psychological outcomes of redefining risk status by testing.

In one study (Wiggins et al. 1992), researchers administered a battery of psychological tests to participants in a pilot testing program for HD. The tests measured levels of psychological distress, depression, and well-being. At each follow-up assessment, the decreased risk group (i.e., those who learned that they did not carry the gene for HD), overall, had lower scores for distress than before testing. The increased risk group showed no significant change from baseline on any measure, although small linear declines appeared in depression and distress. Despite their overall improvement in well-being, however, approximately 10 percent of the *decreased* risk group encountered difficulties in coping with their new status. The good news is no panacea.

Another study (Huggins et al. 1992) outlines the difficulties experienced by six individuals from a *decreased* risk group. Although survivor guilt (i.e., the feeling of "deserting" an affected parent or sibling) was an important factor in the lives of these persons, it was not a major cause of stress or depression. In fact, in this limited sample the individuals most likely to experience adverse effects of learning that they have a decreased risk seemed to be those for whom test results contradicted the outcome of testing that they consciously or unconsciously expected. One man had been unable to make any serious commitments, such as marriage, due to his certainty that he would develop symptoms of HD. Two others who experienced adverse effects had previously made irreversible reproductive decisions (a tubal ligation and a vasectomy). Some participants held unrealistic expectations for the effect of good news on their lives. Huggins et al. speculate that these participants may have believed their quality of life would improve following disclosure, only to suffer disappointment when the good news did not in fact lead to alteration in personal habits and behavior. Although these studies are preliminary, they allow us to conclude that we cannot equate knowledge of a decreased risk status with good news.

In Sarah's case, we are told that the consultand suspects that her test results will be positive. Tempting as it is to assume that forcing the actual results on her would be doing her a favor, an act of justified paternalism, the assumption is problematical.

Forcing test results on Sarah would raise another potential problem. Many counselors feel that it is important to treat all test results in a similar manner, i.e., by giving all test results in person (Quaid 1992). If people with different test results are treated differently, word will get out. People will begin to guess their test results by whether they are asked to return to the center or are given their results over the phone. Differential treatment may have tragic results if a person surmises that he or she carries the HD mutation and acts on that knowledge prior to confirmation and without the benefit of supportive counseling.

Moreover, failure to disclose test results would not impede other family members' access to information about their status. The case indicates that the consultand's children are at risk. However, because we have no information about their ages or their desire to know their gene status, we have insufficient evidence to conclude that Sarah's test results should be disclosed for her children's benefit.

The counselor should not press Sarah's test results on her. One problem with this conclusion is that it may present difficulties for the counselor if Sarah wishes to reconsider learning her test results and seeks further counseling. The counselor would then be in the position of knowing something about the consultand that the consultand has chosen not to know. These circumstances may create a dilemma for the counselor in making choices about the relationship with the consultand, to say nothing of maintaining an affect, tone, and style of objectivity—indeed of ignorance.

One possible solution might be to refer Sarah to another counselor, who has no knowledge of her test results. Even that strategy, however, will not work in all cases: Consultands may prefer to remain with a trusted counselor, and a competent substitute may not be available.

Some counselors have devised ways of minimizing the likelihood of finding themselves in this situation, e.g., by choosing to learn test results only a short time before the consultand appears for discussion of those results. In this case, the counselor learned Sarah's test results seven days before Sarah's scheduled appointment for disclosure. This interval could be shortened significantly if, for example, the counselor adopted the practice of learning test results only twenty-four hours before the appointment. However, that strategy has some drawbacks. It leaves the counselor little time for reflection on the conduct of the disclosure session or double checking laboratory procedures and results. Moreover, it can only reduce—not completely eliminate—the possibility that the counselor will know the test results if and when the consultand changes his or her mind about receiving results.

In the end, however, our conclusion in this case is clear. The counselor should not take the initiative in contacting Sarah; Sarah has a right to change her mind. She should be told her test results only if she asks for them.

Case 4 Ann and Jack

In late 1990, before direct gene testing for HD was available, two siblings, Ann and Jack, requested predictive testing. They are in their thirties; Jack is married. Mr. Roberts, their father, had been diagnosed with HD at age 58, although there was no previous family history of the disorder. His father, Ann and Jack's Grandfather Roberts, had died at the age of 92 with no psychiatric or motor symptoms, but as part of their father's work-up a blood sample had been banked from Grandfather Roberts. Their paternal grandmother had died in her thirties; all of her siblings had died relatively young. Mr. Roberts, however, had two sisters, Gladys, 74, and Lila, 68, who were unaffected. Samples and medical records were obtained from Gladys and Lila in order to recreate Grandmother Roberts's haplotype. The availability of a blood sample from their unaffected grandfather enabled linkage testing.

Because Mr. Roberts's HD had been diagnosed in the absence of a previous family history of the disorder, paternity testing was done. The results indicated that Mr. Roberts, Gladys, and Lila were indeed the children of Grandfather Roberts.

During pretest counseling, the counselor carefully explained to Ann and Jack that the likelihood that Grandfather Roberts carried the gene for HD was very small. The linkage analysis assumed that the HD gene was inherited from their Grandmother Roberts, about whom little was known. Ann and Jack were aware of the uncertainties of testing, but they decided that even some information would be better than their current situation, and they both decided to proceed.

Linkage testing indicated that both Jack and Ann had inherited from their father the chromosome 4 that he had inherited from his unaffected father. Ann and Jack were told that their risk for developing HD was low; the counselor stressed the uncertainties and assumptions of linkage testing as well as the uncertainties based on their unclear family history.

Two years later, a neurologist called the testing center to request predictive testing for one of his patients, who turned out to be Ann and

Jack's Aunt Lila. The neurologist explained that Lila, now 68 years old, wanted to clarify her risk of HD for her two children once and for all. The neurologist assured the testing center that Lila was not showing any symptoms. The center scheduled a neurological exam for Lila as a first step in the testing protocol.

Lila was seen in clinic several weeks later. The center neurologist felt that she was showing early, but definite, symptoms of HD and shared his diagnosis with Lila and her husband. Based on this new information, the counselor again looked at the results of the linkage test performed two years earlier. A comparison of the linkage results of Lila and her affected brother indicated that the chromosome 4 that they shared was the one that they had inherited from their unaffected father. The counselor was uncertain how to interpret this finding; one possible explanation was crossover during meiosis. In any case, she did not share the information with any other family members.

In March 1993, the gene for HD was found, enabling direct gene testing for HD. The laboratory at the university where the counselor worked was now preparing to offer direct gene testing. The lab director offered to run the first fifty samples free of charge, assigning first priority to individuals who had been previously tested through linkage. The lab director agreed to run samples of persons at risk and their closest affected relative. The lab director asked the counselor for a list of the sample numbers of these individuals. Due to the uncertain history in Ann and Jack's case, and the new information about intermediate alleles discovered after the gene was found, the counselor included the sample number of the grandfather on this list.

The counselor then sent letters to all individuals who had been tested using linkage to ask whether they would like their samples rerun using direct gene testing and, if so, to obtain their consent. The letter stressed the possibility of error inherent in the linkage process and the possibility that some results could be reversed. Ann and Jack, satisfied with their results, both declined repeat testing.

In the meantime, the laboratory had tested the samples on the list. The test results revealed that Ann and Jack's grandfather had 32 and 39 CAG repeats. In effect, he had an intermediate allele, which had expanded into the HD range in their father. Their father's repeat sizes were 19 and 42. As Ann and Jack had the chromosome 4 that their father had inherited from his father, it was obvious that both Ann and Jack had inherited the HD mutation from their father; in fact their repeat sizes were 17 and 43, and 18 and 44, respectively.

The counselor was extremely upset. She now had important infor-

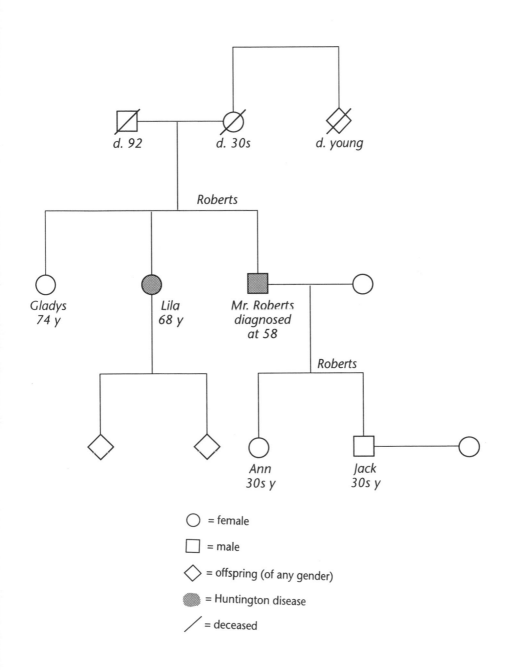

d. 92   d. 30s   d. young

Roberts

Gladys   Lila   Mr. Roberts
74 y   68 y   diagnosed
                           at 58

Roberts

Ann   Jack
30s y   30s y

◯ = female

▢ = male

◇ = offspring (of any gender)

⬤ = Huntington disease

╱ = deceased

*mation about Ann and Jack that they did not wish to know, but that had
serious ramifications for them and their families.*

This case raises issues on two levels. One issue concerns the direct gene
testing of Ann and Jack's DNA—the process through which the counselor has acquired the "upsetting" information. The second question
concerns what she should do now that she has the information.

The Ramifications of Direct Testing

It is not difficult to make the case that the counselor should not
have this information at all. The purpose of rerunning the samples was
to check the reliability of the laboratory. We assume that the terms of
Mr. Roberts's original consent to donate allow for this corroborative
step. The laboratory received only the sample numbers; it ran the samples blind. Thus, only the counselor knew the status (affected or unaffected) of each person who had contributed a sample, and only the counselor was able to check the accuracy of direct gene testing against linkage
results. The inevitable result, when a reversal appeared, is the present dilemma. The situation could have been avoided by blinding the counselor but not the laboratory. Samples could have been chosen at random
and the results of the linkage analysis attached, so that the counselor—
although not the laboratory—would remain blind to the results of the
trial run. In contrast, if the results of individuals' tests are revealed to the
counselor, we seem to have moved from an exercise in checking laboratory procedures into a *second* clinical test.

Would it be legitimate to run a second test without the consent of
Ann and Jack? A majority of us feels it was wrong to submit the samples
without prior consent of the individuals involved, i.e., that consent for
direct gene testing should have been secured before the list was given to
the laboratory.

A minority opposes this conclusion, arguing that Ann and Jack's
original consent should be construed broadly—not simply as a consent
to a specific procedure but as a consent to make optimal use of their
DNA samples to determine their risk for HD. Linkage testing assigned
risk on the basis of segregation of markers near the HD gene; with the
advent of direct gene testing, the gene itself is identified. Ann and Jack's
current refusal of additional testing is compromised by the fact that they
have been given an erroneous test result.

These arguments leave the majority unmoved. They argue that the
original consent was quite specific, that it was given two years ago, and
that—whatever misinformation they may have—Ann and Jack are now

clearly competent and have opted out of confirmatory testing. These arguments suggest that the samples should not have been retested, at least not in any way in which the results of the tests could affect their clinical care.

What to Do Now?

Ann and Jack have been asked if they want to be retested, and they have said no. This situation leaves three possibilities. The counselor may do nothing, inform Ann and Jack of the results of the direct test, or take steps to make sure that they rethink their decision.

There is a good argument for doing nothing beyond sending the letter that has already been sent to individuals previously tested with linkage analysis, especially if one takes the view that the samples should not have been retested without a second consent. As one member of our group put it, "Doing nothing comes as close as possible to recreating the moral universe as it would be if the mistake had never happened." After all, Ann and Jack have been asked if they want further information, and they have declined. Doing nothing honors their latest choice, which is to decline to learn more about their risk. Of course, this argument assumes that the contact inviting them to participate in retesting—whether it be a letter or clinical visit—is not pro forma but seriously raises the possibility that the earlier testing may have been mistaken. A majority of our group favors this course of action.

The second option, an extreme alternative, would be to assume that the original consent controlled, and to inform Ann and Jack straightaway that they carry the HD gene. None of us favors this course. Not only would this verbal assault ignore the reality of the second consent, but even if that consent were unnecessary—or if it had not been requested—the counselor would be mistaken to tell Ann and Jack the results of direct testing without seeking to determine whether they *now* want it. Two years have passed; Ann and Jack are certainly somewhat changed, and their life circumstances may have altered. If a mistake in linkage were to be discovered forty-eight hours after the fact, it is arguable that the consultand's misperceptions should be corrected immediately. But that is not this case.

The third option, favored by a small minority, holds that the counselor has a special duty to challenge Ann and Jack's tragically mistaken sense of security. The center has seriously, if inadvertently, misinformed Ann and Jack, who chose testing when they believed themselves to be at 50 percent risk. Their decision to refuse confirmatory testing cannot be abstracted from its context: They believe that the odds are 90 percent or better that they do not have the HD gene. Their current decision making is encumbered by this misperception; we cannot know how they would now feel if we were to revert to the status quo and a supposed risk factor of 50 percent.

The minority holds that the counselor has a responsibility to shake Ann and Jack's sense of security without disclosing the results of the direct test. This goal might be accomplished in two ways. First, if Aunt Lila will agree to make her diagnosis known, this specific information can be used to suggest to Ann and Jack the precariousness of the linkage results in their family. Second, the issue can be raised with them a second time—after the first letter—in a focused way. If they refuse direct testing after one or another of these probings, their refusal should be respected. If they choose testing, they should be asked for another sample, and a confirmatory test should be run.

That is a minority view. Our majority feels that Ann and Jack have been given sufficient opportunity to change their minds. Whatever mistakes may have been made in the past, they provide no justification for further intrusions in these people's lives.

Case 5 *Carol*

Carol, a thirty-nine-year-old woman, donated a tissue sample as part of a linkage study of BRCA1 in her extended family. All three of her older sisters have been diagnosed with either breast or ovarian cancer. Her oldest sister was diagnosed with ovarian cancer at age forty-seven; her other two sisters developed breast cancer at ages forty-two and forty-five. Results of Carol's linkage test show that Carol herself is not at risk. Carol made it clear she did not want to know test results, although the opportunity to receive that information was offered to her when she donated her sample. She contemplates a prophylactic bilateral mastectomy and oophorectomy. She has a twelve-year-old daughter, Jenny. Should Carol be told her test results?

In this case we have a woman who agreed to participate in a research project but did not want to know the study results. Because she declined before results were obtained, a counselor at the study center can contact Carol and offer her the opportunity to receive her test results. If she declines again, the counselor need not take further action. It is important to keep in mind that the counselor probably will be calling all of the families who participated in research to advise them that the BRCA1 gene has been isolated and that direct gene testing will be available in the future. Thus, Carol probably will have another opportunity to receive accurate results.

We explored a similar "refusal of results" case for Huntington disease in Case 3, "Sarah." Most of the issues discussed in that case apply here with the following exception: Data support the fact that when women have a better understanding of their "true" risk versus a "perceived" risk, the information generally enhances health-promoting behavior, i.e., breast self-exam and mammography (Kash 1992). Linkage analysis has determined that Carol does not carry the gene predisposing to breast cancer in her family. Still, she has an approximate lifetime risk of one in eight of developing breast cancer, the risk of breast cancer in the general population. In contrast to HD, negative linkage results do not mean she will not develop the disease; the finding simply means that her risk is lower than that of her sisters, who we assume are gene carriers. Despite the potential for engaging this woman in health-promoting behavior based on accurate risk results, Carol's negative test results should not compel the counselor to override the consultand's wishes.

As noted in the discussion of Case 3, "Sarah," Huggins et al. (1992) found that one of the predictors of distress experienced by the "good news" group was test results that contradicted the individual's conscious or unconscious expectations. They offered the example of persons who had made an irreversible surgical decision such as vasectomy or tubal ligation. If Carol had already undergone prophylactic oophorectomy and mastectomy because of her family history, she would be a perfect candidate to suffer adverse effects from learning her linkage results. As the only one of four female siblings who did not inherit a BRCA1 mutation, she may also be an ideal candidate for survivor guilt. Even if those were the facts, the promise to respect her choice not to know should be kept.

The case as written offers no compelling argument for the counselor to disclose results based on Carol's contemplation of surgery. She should explore Carol's thoughts regarding disease, risk, and prophylactic surgery and strongly advise Carol to learn her test results prior to surgery. That can be done without indirectly disclosing results. In this situation, Carol clearly would benefit from being informed of her gene status. Furthermore, it is difficult to imagine any woman declining information that might spare her from bilateral mastectomies, let alone oophorectomy. Significant morbidity and even mortality are associated with each of these surgical procedures.

What if Carol insists on surgery? Would a surgeon be obligated to obtain the genetic test results prior to performing the procedures? What if Carol doesn't inform the surgeon of the existence of the research study? Should he simply look at her family pedigree, calculate her risk, and agree to her request? Should he obtain a second opinion, and from whom? Testing for the BRCA1 gene is obviously relevant to the wisdom of a choice for surgery, and the surgeon has a responsibility to learn whether a test for BRCA1 has been done and, if so, its result. Before performing radical surgery, a surgeon should document familial cancer or refer the patient to a genetic counseling center familiar with assessment of cancer risk to support the request for prophylactic surgery.

At age twelve, Carol's daughter Jenny probably was not a part of the linkage study. She would be highly unlikely to develop cancer now or in the next several years, even if she were a gene carrier (which, in all probability, she is not). After three of her aunts have developed the disease, she is probably aware of breast and ovarian cancer in her family. If she has cousins, she may well have discussed the issue with them. The case does not indicate that Jenny wants to be tested, and there is no medical reason to test her now, certainly not absent her request.

On the other hand, Carol has responsibilities to Jenny that the counselor should explore with her. If Jenny is anxious about the possibility that her developing body will become a target for cancer, Carol should help her. At a minimum, Carol should contact the counseling center to inform herself about the genetics of BRCA1 and Jenny's calculated risk at age twelve. This information need not include disclosure of Carol's own test results.

Some argue that Carol should be willing to learn her result for Jenny's sake, but knowledge of Carol's negative test results might not liberate Jenny from continued anxiety. One study (Lynch 1993) documented disbelief among younger women who were told they were not gene carriers. These gene-negative individuals maintained a state of anxiety regarding cancer development. They indicated that they would continue intense surveillance and would still consider prophylactic surgery. Carol needs to be aware of these possibilities and alert to signs that Jenny remains anxious and worried. If Jenny is distressed, Carol should know that therapeutic counseling may be helpful.

Case 6 *Kirsten and David*

Kirsten is a twenty-nine-year-old woman whose husband, David, is at 50 percent risk for HD. She contacts a predictive testing center, reporting that she has discovered she is six weeks pregnant and wants to have the fetus tested for the HD mutation. In a counseling session, Kirsten and David reveal that the pregnancy is unplanned and that David is undecided about whether he wants the predictive test for himself. Kirsten, however, feels very strongly that she does not want their child to be at any risk for HD. Now that the technology is available, she wants to use it to enable her to decide whether to continue the pregnancy.

Kirsten is aware that a positive prenatal result would reveal that David has the HD mutation. Nondisclosing prenatal exclusion testing (see Glossary) is not an option, as both of David's parents are deceased.

Kirsten insists that she be allowed to proceed with prenatal testing. David, however, does not feel prepared emotionally for the possibility of receiving two positive results at once and then proceeding with a termination of the pregnancy. He believes they should continue the pregnancy. He believes that if the baby is a gene carrier, preventive treatment will be available by the time he or she is an adult.

This case poses questions about the ethical obligations of the counselor and both parties to the marriage.

Counselor

The law gives Kirsten a constitutional right to seek an abortion in certain circumstances and precludes her husband, David, from exercising a veto over her choice (*Planned Parenthood v. Casey*). However, the law does not require anyone to perform an abortion or to provide information to help a woman decide whether to terminate a pregnancy (*Poelker v. Doe*). Therefore, the counselor is not obligated by *Roe v. Wade* or subsequent cases to provide prenatal testing for Kirsten. The question is what the counselor *ought* to do, not what the law requires her to do.

Here the counselor has established a relationship with both Kirsten and David. Thus, she owes both of them an obligation to act as a fiduciary, that is, with the utmost good faith and in their best interests. Unfortunately, the best interests of the spouses appear to conflict. Standard pro-choice rhetoric suggests that the woman's interest always outweighs the man's because she experiences the greater impact of pregnancy and childbirth. Standard right-to-life rhetoric argues that a fetus's right to be born outweighs a woman's right to choose; in this case, that line of reasoning may lead to a decision to refrain from testing, as the husband prefers.

Neither position is helpful here. The impact on David of learning that he carries the HD gene (and even the impact of denying him control over what he learns about his own health) means that he has a greater stake in the decision than male partners in more typical abortion situations. Moreover, many persons who do not oppose abortion rights for women continue to believe that men should have a significant role in deciding whether a pregnancy should be terminated. On the other hand, Kirsten clearly has the power to end her pregnancy, and refusing to test may lead her to obtain an abortion if she thinks there is any risk of bearing a child who carries the HD mutation. Thus, although we cannot predict what she will do, it is possible that refusing prenatal testing will actually increase the probability of abortion, even the abortion of a fetus that does not carry the HD mutation.

Obviously, the counselor should work with the couple to try to resolve the disagreement. Kirsten is only six weeks pregnant. This gives the counselor four to ten weeks to help the couple reach a consensus. (Chorionic villus sampling is routinely performed between ten and thirteen weeks of gestation, early amniocentesis at thirteen to fourteen weeks, and regular amniocentesis at sixteen to twenty weeks.) That time may be especially important in a case like this one, where one wonders about the quality of communication within the marriage.

The facts of the case leave Kirsten's situation vague. Whereas David has known of his risk for some time, she may have learned of it only recently, and she has known of the pregnancy for only about a month. She may not grasp what her insistence on testing the fetus says to David. Sound counseling practice includes efforts to help consultands understand the full ramifications of their actions and to make truly informed decisions. Nonetheless, counseling may fail to resolve the disagreement. If that happens, the counselor will have to decide whether to make testing available.

In reaching a decision, the counselor will not be helped much by considering the interests of the fetus because those interests (if any) are

unclear. We distinguish fetal interest from the interest of the unconceived, which we dismiss as speculative and irrelevant in Case 1, "Paul
and Michael." In this case, it is difficult to know whether the fetus's interest is in having a life or in avoiding the suffering of HD or of being at
risk for HD. Thirty-five years of healthy existence may seem an unmixed
blessing. However, Farrer (1986) found that the rate of suicide for persons diagnosed with HD is four times that of the U.S. Caucasian population, and Schoenfeld et al. (1984) also found an elevated suicide risk in
persons diagnosed with or suspected of having HD. We lack the ability
to compare the benefits of thirty-five years of good health with the suffering of fifteen years after diagnosis with HD.

Are there other outside factors or interests to consider? In Case 1,
"Paul and Michael," we argued that allowing a person in a position of
power to consider general societal interests is problematic. However, this
case differs from Case 1 in that here the counselor has conflicting obligations to two persons with whom she has established a professional relationship. If the two consultands' interests are equally strong, the counselor must find a way to resolve the impasse between Kirsten and David.
In these circumstances, appealing to broader social values is not running
roughshod over an individual for the good of the society; it is setting a
tragic choice in a larger and somewhat particularized social context.

Here the background value of relevance is our society's investment
in genetic counseling programs. The raison d'etre of genetic testing programs is to maximize informed consultand decision making. Ethical considerations may sometimes suggest that individual consultands should
not be tested and surely will make us reluctant to consider requiring testing. When professionals offer a service that society has decided is worth-
while, they should provide that service to all who seek it unless a strong
reason to withhold the service can be shown. Genetic counseling, however, should be available to all to facilitate informed decision making.
The burden of proof is on a decision not to test; as in Case 1, "Paul and
Michael," we conclude that David's choice to refuse to learn his risk cannot outweigh Kirsten's claim to informed choices about her reproductive life.

Kirsten and David

As parties to a marriage, Kirsten and David should work to resolve
their differences. Indeed, one could argue that this couple should have
addressed this situation long before the present crisis arose. Nonetheless, they apparently have not done so, and the question of their ethical
obligations if they are unable to reach agreement must be addressed.

Consistent with our advocacy of referral to appropriate professionals, we think it would be appropriate for the counselor to refer this couple for marriage counseling. (See Guideline IIIC.)

Trying to find an ethical obligation for David to undergo testing has some appeal. David is a moral agent, not the helpless subject of a search for information like the fetus. If David is free of the HD mutation, the need for prenatal testing will be eliminated. Indeed, one member of our group thinks that David owes his spouse an ethical obligation to be tested. However, the majority thinks that argument goes too far. Testing David reduces the possibility that the fetus will have to be tested only by 50 percent. (If David tests positive—a 50 percent chance—the fetus will still have to be tested.) Moreover, testing is repugnant to David. His freedom to refuse to be tested sharpens the issue for Kirsten and forces her to decide just how serious she is about learning the information; it forecloses a possible cheap way out for her. When she is pursuing a course with the grave implications involved here, it is desirable to ensure that the decision she confronts is a difficult one.

Ultimately, if Kirsten continues to seek prenatal testing, we do not think it is unethical for her to obtain it. She has obligations to herself and an obligation to exercise her best judgment on behalf of the fetus, as well as obligations to David. Her resolution of her competing obligations seems to be the kind of decision about which reasonable persons can disagree. Therefore, we cannot justify condemning any choice she makes. For all we know, Kirsten may choose abortion if she does not succeed in obtaining testing. If the alternative to being tested turns out to be the abortion of a fetus who may be healthy, the decision not to be tested may be more problematic than the decision to be tested.

Another option would be to carry the pregnancy to term and give birth to a child whose HD status is unknown. However, we see no reason to insist that that is Kirsten's only ethical option. The availability of prenatal testing provides the opportunity for persons to exercise judgments based on information that otherwise would not be available. The choice to obtain that information cannot be condemned, at least not on the facts of this case.

Case 7 Robert

Robert, the father of two young adult daughters, requests predictive genetic testing for autosomal dominant polycystic kidney disease (ADPKD). After watching his mother die of ADPKD before dialysis and transplantation were widely available, he is anxious about his own health and wishes to know his genetic status.

The first of his children, born twenty-five years ago, died days after birth from polycystic kidney disease. An infant cousin had been similarly affected and died many years before. Despite the knowledge that several adults in the extended family (including Robert's mother) suffered from the autosomal dominant form of the disease, physicians at the time diagnosed the two infants with the recessive form of polycystic kidney disease. It was thought that infants could not be affected by the dominant form of PKD, and the physicians informed the family that the presence of both forms of PKD in the family was coincidental. In reading the current literature, however, Robert is surprised to learn that it is now recognized that infants can indeed be affected by ADPKD and that his first child probably died of the dominant form of the disorder.

Robert's test results reveal that he does carry the gene for ADPKD. He refuses to inform his daughters, both of whom plan to have children soon, about his test results. Robert explains this choice by saying that he thinks insurance difficulties for them are a more serious problem than awareness of possible health risks during pregnancy or the opportunity for them to make personal decisions related to carrying or perpetuating the ADPKD gene. Neither of Robert's daughters is a client of the genetic counselor.

The issue in this case is whether an individual has the moral right to withhold information about himself when that information has direct relevance for the health and reproductive choices of his adult children. As a corollary, is a health care professional justified in breaching the consultand's confidentiality and disclosing information to first-degree relatives without the consultand's consent?

Robert has just learned that he carries the gene for ADPKD, which means that each of his two adult daughters has a 50 percent chance of having inherited the ADPKD gene. The narrative of the case leaves an important question unanswered: whether the daughters are aware of their family history of ADPKD. Do they know the cause of their grandmother's death? If they do, and if the genetics of the condition have been explained to them, then they would be aware of their own 25 percent risk and, perhaps, the possibility of direct gene testing regardless of their father's actions. The amount of information they have is a fact of great relevance.

Our first analysis assumes that they know nothing about the condition in their family. Some argue that genetics professionals should be legally permitted to disclose such relevant information to relatives at risk (Wertz and Fletcher 1988). However, not all relatives either desire or appreciate this information (Quaid 1992; Wexler 1992). Sharing highly personal medical information that involves reproduction and future health can raise troubling emotional and practical issues, which may lead an individual diagnosed with a genetic disease to withhold relevant health information from other family members, thereby denying them the option of seeking testing (Andrews et al. 1994). While most counselors agree that consultands should be encouraged to inform relatives about pertinent genetic information, disclosure of information to those relatives without the consent of the consultand is much more controversial and can be justified only in rare circumstances.

What are these circumstances? In Case 6, "Kirsten and David," we briefly touched on whether spouses have a right to know the genetic status of their husbands or wives. In that case we argued that a husband's choice not to determine his genetic status was not a sufficient reason to deny his pregnant wife prenatal testing. However, we did not discuss the counselor's responsibilities to a spouse who was unaware of the risk, nor did we resolve the issue of whether a spouse has a right to learn the results of a test that has already been performed.

An argument may be made that blood relatives have a more convincing claim than spouses to the results of a genetic test that may have implications for their own lives. However, in Case 2, "Father and Son," we concluded that it was difficult if not impossible to generalize in terms of type of relationship. In a 1990 survey, a majority of geneticists in the United States (58 percent) said that they would breach confidentiality and disclose genetic information concerning a risk for HD to an unsuspecting relative without the patient's permission and even over the patient's refusal (Wertz et al. 1990). Factors that might strengthen the case for disclosure include (1) a reasonable, yet unsuccessful, attempt has been made to elicit voluntary disclosure; (2) there is a high likelihood that the relative has the genetic defect; (3) the defect presents a serious risk to the relative; and (4) there is reason to believe that the disclosure is necessary to prevent serious harm (President's Commission 1983).

With this background in mind, the counselor's first approach should be to try to convince Robert to reveal his test results to his daughters. Although they may lose needed insurance coverage, that risk seems less significant than the fact that each daughter is currently at 50 percent risk for a serious disease. Robert's refusal to share his test results denies them the chance to decide for themselves what value they place on possible insurance loss as opposed to their own health and the health of children they may have. Being informed of Robert's test results would enable each of his daughters to monitor her own health, consider testing for herself, or consider prenatal testing, if her test reveals that she carries the ADPKD gene. Thus, disclosure would aid Robert's daughters in making decisions about their own health care at this moment and in planning for the future health of possible children.

Some may think that this approach violates the principles of nondirective counseling, but we maintain that a counselor should be encouraged to explore the consequences of a consultand's choice with the consultand. (See Arras 1990.) In this case, the outcomes to be considered include the possibility that Robert's daughters may already have symptoms of ADPKD that require treatment but might not be found without information regarding the family history; his daughters' reactions should they find out about their risk only after having children; and the possibility that one of his grandchildren might have the juvenile form of ADPKD. We think that Robert must at least contemplate these serious consequences.

The counselor should also be sensitive to the nuances of the case. Robert has only recently learned that the death of his baby daughter many years before was probably directly related to her inheriting the ADPKD gene from him. This new knowledge may be emotionally overwhelming, as Robert attempts to deal with his own health concerns and potential guilt about the death of his daughter. It may be his sense of shame and guilt, rather than the actual outcome of his test, that he wishes to protect. The counselor should be willing to explore this possibility with Robert.

The majority of people in Robert's situation eventually share their genetic information with relatives at risk (personal communication, Kimberly A. Quaid). As Robert comes to terms with the new knowledge that he is a gene carrier, it is likely that he will choose to reveal this information to his daughters.

What if Robert declines to disclose his genetic status to his daughters, however? People in general are morally obliged to help a readily identifiable person whose need is great when the burden of helping is small. Wertz and Fletcher have argued that medical caregivers' obligation to warn third parties of harm should trump their obligation to protect patient confidentiality if a patient refuses to inform siblings or children that they are at risk of HD. They assert that professionals must "seek out and inform the unsuspecting" (Wertz and Fletcher 1989b, 222), opting for disclosure in order to provide family members with full information about their own future.

In this case the information about Robert's genetic status is clearly relevant to the daughters, they are easily accessible, and they may regard their father's reasons for refusing to disclose as relatively insubstantial. If they are unaware that they are at risk, the counselor must be sure that they receive that information, by breaking confidentiality if necessary.

On the other hand, the counselor does not have a professional relationship with either of Robert's daughters. Absent such a relationship, it is difficult to argue that the counselor has either a legal duty to warn these young women or a duty to break Robert's confidentiality *if they already know themselves to be at risk*. (See Case 8, "Mr. H.") The case for breaching Robert's confidentiality is much weaker than in Case 11, "Maurice," in which an airline pilot who carries the HD mutation may put innocent persons at risk. Robert is doing nothing of the kind. The magnitude of the risk is radically different, and he is not causing the risk in anything like the same sense of the word *cause*.

The justification for breaching confidentiality turns on what Robert's daughters know. If they already know they are at risk, breach of confidentiality to shift the odds from 25 percent to 50 percent is unjustified; if they do not know they are at risk, the breach is justified. (See Cases 5, "Carol," and 10, "Mary Ann.")

Our minority rejects this distinction in terms of knowledge of risk, holding that everything turns on the magnitude of harms and benefit to the concerned persons. In this case, they claim that a breach of confidentiality is justified; judgments about other cases would entirely depend on the facts in those situations.

In sum: Robert's daughters are entitled to know that they are at risk for a serious genetic disease, but not necessarily to know the results of their father's test for ADPKD. We believe that Robert should tell them both the family history and the results of his test, and that the counselor should advise him accordingly. If they know nothing of the family history, and if Robert refuses to inform them that they are at risk, the counselor should breach confidentiality and tell them that they are at risk.

Case 8 Mr. H.

A neurologist requested confirmatory testing of Huntington disease in Mr. H., a man in the late stages of the disease. Mr. H. has five children ranging in age from late teens to mid-twenties, and two grandchildren. One of his children, John H., delivered his father's blood sample and asked about the accuracy of the testing for Mr. H. and presymptomatic testing for his children. At the time, John H. said that none of the children wanted to pursue testing because of career and insurance concerns. DNA testing of Mr. H's sample confirmed the presence of alleles in the affected and "gray zone," 41 and 36 CAG repeats, respectively.

Family history revealed that Mr. H.'s father had HD. His mother's family had no history of HD; she died in her eighties, reportedly of natural causes. The testing program informed the neurologist that DNA testing had detected an abnormality consistent with HD but did not reveal the sizes of the two alleles or that the risk of Mr. H's children inheriting the gene may be not 50 percent but closer to 100 percent. Because John H. had stated that the children did not want to know their status yet, this information was not reported.

The testing program debated first, whether nondisclosure of repeat length was the best course of action and, second, what should be done in the event that any of the proband's children request testing.

It is now known that HD is associated with a repeating and unstable CAG trinucleotide on chromosome 4. (See Introduction and Glossary.) Earlier, HD was thought to be inherited as a completely penetrant gene. That is, if an individual inherited the gene, he or she would inevitably develop the disease. However, the discovery of a range of repeats has clouded that certainty, creating some confusion about the precise number of repeats (CAG_n) required to cause HD. An emerging consensus is as follows:

26 and below = normal
27–35 repeats = nonpenetrant with meiotic instability

36–39 repeats = variably penetrant with meiotic instability
40 and above = HD (ACMG/ASHG Huntington Disease Genetic Testing Working Group 1998).

Even though the CAG repeat length is highly sensitive and specific for predicting whether someone will develop HD at some time in the future, the expected age of onset cannot be predicted with certainty. In general, CAG repeat length only accounts for 50 percent of the variation in age of onset (Andrew et al. 1993, Duyao et al. 1993, Snell et al. 1993). Limited ability to predict age of onset has led many testing centers to adopt a policy of withholding disclosure of repeat length, instead conveying test results categorically (Duyao et al. 1993, Benjamin et al. 1994, Huntington Study Group 1994). Other authors insist that individuals may have a right to choose to know this information (Burgess and Hayden 1996).

Mr. H., the affected proband in this case, was found to have alleles with 41 and 36 CAG repeats, which effectively diagnoses him with HD but creates uncertainty for his children. Any of his children who have inherited the paternal allele with 41 CAG repeats could be informed with confidence that they will develop HD. If they inherit the allele with 36 repeats, however, it is not clear whether they will develop HD. Their paternal grandmother (from whom their father presumably inherited the allele with 36 repeats) lived into her eighties, apparently without showing symptoms of the disorder, but the case does not provide genetic information about her. Moreover, the intermediate allele that the proband inherited from his mother may expand during spermatogenesis from 36 repeats, increasing the likelihood that that allele also will cause HD in his offspring. Expansion is more likely to occur when the HD gene is paternally transmitted (MacDonald et al. 1993; Telenius et al. 1994). One study reports that in a small series of cases, the likelihood that an intermediate allele would expand into the HD range is 42 percent (Goldberg et al. 1993). Thus, the researchers reason that the risk of HD for Mr. H's children exceeds 50 percent and may be as high as 70 percent.

The testing center has fulfilled the letter of its obligation by confirming Mr. H's diagnosis of HD. However, the center limited the information in its report to the specific question asked by the neurologist. The staff describes concern about the appropriateness of "nondisclosure of repeat length" (the proband's CAG_n).

The testing center should determine the purpose of the neurologist's request for confirmatory testing in Mr. H. The goals of testing might be to rule out another neurological disorder and to provide accurate information to Mr. H's children regarding their risk of HD should they request that information at some later time. It appears that Mr. H's diagnosis is not in question. His father died of HD, and the case does not describe any uncertainty about his diagnosis. The testing center should provide full and accurate test results, including allele sizes, to the neurologist.

A second question for the testing center concerns what to do if Mr. H's children request testing. We believe that the children should be informed that the recent testing has revealed new information about their father's status and ask them whether they wish to be informed about the results and their implications. Mr. H's diagnosis is well established, and there is no reason to suppose that he would object to their learning the full details of his test results. (Compare Case 27, "Aunt Mary.") The children already know that they are at risk of developing HD; the only uncertainty is the odds. Consistent with our argument in Case 3, "Sarah," they should not be given information that they choose not to know.

Results that reveal uncertain risk, as in this case, may impose difficult situations on patients who seek a resolution to uncertainty and also for counselors, who wish to provide clear and definitive information on which their consultands can act. These ambiguous results may be particularly agonizing with the advent of direct gene testing. In contrast to linkage analysis, which at best could at best provide only probabilities, direct gene testing held out the promise of a definitive answer to the question of whether an individual would or would not develop HD. The discovery of the previously unsuspected "gray zone" actually may leave some patients worse off in terms of assurance about their future. (See Case 4, "Ann and Jack.")

This conclusion has implications for a wide range of genetic disorders. Before the discovery of the "gray zone," HD appeared to be unique in its complete penetrance and expressivity. The more common case is variability, which may be even more marked in disorders with incomplete penetrance and polygenic disorders. Unfortunately, counselors and patients must continue to live with uncertainty. It would be scientifically irresponsible and morally wrong to make exaggerated claims for the ability of genetic testing to resolve difficult human quandaries.

Case 9 Natalie

Natalie, a thirty-five-year-old woman whose father has HD, requested predictive testing for herself. DNA samples had been previously banked for both her mother and father. As part of a research study to clarify the inheritance of the HD gene and the number of CAG repeats, both of these samples were rerun along with Natalie's at her request. The laboratory results indicated that while Natalie had 17 and 19 CAG repeats, Natalie's mother, Helen, had 17 and 39 CAG repeats. These results were surprising, given the fact that Helen came from a family with no history of HD. The testing center informed Natalie of these results and their implications for the possibility of Helen's developing HD. Natalie asked the testing center not to share this information with Helen; she was consumed with taking care of Natalie's father, who was still at home and in the later stages of the disease. Natalie felt that the information would be emotionally devastating to her mother. This information also had ramifications for Natalie's two brothers, who had explicitly stated that they were not interested in testing. The counselor now knew that the risk to each of these brothers was 75 percent, without taking account of the mother's age, rather than 50 percent, as previously thought, and debated whether this information should be conveyed to them.

The results of testing to date show that Natalie's CAG_n is below the range associated with HD, indicating that she will not develop the disorder. Her mother, however, who was previously assumed not to be at risk, is now known not only to be at risk, but almost certainly a carrier of the mutation. One group reports that approximately 1 in 150 samples from individuals from the general population who are not at risk reveal an intermediate HD allele (Kremer et al. 1994). Nonetheless, Helen's test results seem so surprising that the first course of action should probably be to determine whether the results are wrong. If possible, her sample should be rerun. If it cannot be rerun, or if the possibility exists that the sample has been contaminated or mislabeled, then the issue of obtaining a new sample will arise. Some disingenuousness is involved if the center asks for a new sample while saying only that it is needed because of a possible problem with the first sample. That disingenuousness is probably tolerable, however, given the modesty of the physical invasion and the serious risk of upsetting Helen by revealing the real reason for requesting the new sample.

If reevaluation confirms Helen's results, then the questions will arise of whether to disclose her risk to her and what to tell her sons.

Helen

Preliminary Issues

In order to resolve this case, we should know what Helen was told and what she agreed to at the time she provided her sample. If she chose to receive no information about her own status, then none should be conveyed to her now. For all we know, she might have been unwilling to provide a sample if she had thought that doing so might lead to her learning unwanted information about herself.

This case highlights a problem that arises in many contexts. Clinicians and researchers often fail to consider the possibility of learning unsought or unexpected information in the course of genetic testing. The frequency of this problem, however, suggests that the possibility should be a routine consideration in genetic testing. As part of the informed consent process, patients and research subjects should be informed about the possibility that unexpected information will be discovered, and informed consent should cover disclosure or nondisclosure of such information.

It would also be useful to know Helen's age. While her age alone might not resolve the question of whether to tell her the new findings, the older she is, the less likely it is that she will develop HD. A reduced probability that she will be affected both weakens the case for disclosure and suggests that if disclosure is made, it can be accompanied by truthful counseling that downplays the significance of the new information for Helen.

In the case of an intermediate allele, however, age might not be all that significant. One of the problems in conveying information about repeats in the 36-to-39 range is that the literature shows individuals with 39 repeats who have mild symptoms in their eighties, no symptoms in their nineties, and other variations. With a CAG repeat of 39, it is not possible to predict whether Helen will show symptoms. Standard probability and risk assessments based on an average age of onset of thirty-eight or thirty-nine simply do not apply in such cases. Our analysis proceeds on the assumption that no agreement about disclosure of results was made when Helen provided her sample, and we make no assumption about Helen's age other than recognizing that she is old enough to have a thirty-five-year-old daughter.

Another part of the ethical dilemma in this case is caused by ethically problematic conduct that has already occurred. Natalie sought predictive testing for herself. Her diagnosis was not affected by her mother's status. Therefore, information about Helen should not have been given to Natalie. If an appropriate course of conduct had been followed, the counselor would now be able to make a professional and ethical judgment about what to tell Helen, free of the confusion raised by Natalie's possibly unreliable account of her mother's condition. Nonetheless, this analysis will deal with the situation as it actually is, rather than as it should have been.

Analysis

If the issue here is defined as whether to disclose information to Helen, the case is a difficult one. Some factors make it a weaker and some factors make it a stronger case for disclosure than others we have seen. On the one hand, because no public health or safety issue is at stake here, the case for disclosure is weaker than in Case 11, "Maurice." It is also weaker than in Case 10, "Mary Ann," because Helen cannot use the new information to engage in potentially lifesaving behavior. On the other hand, Natalie has no confidentiality claim because the relevant information is not about her. Therefore, if we see this as a case about whether to disclose information, the proper resolution is unclear. Moreover, characterizing it as a disclosure-nondisclosure case ignores the value of Helen's freedom of choice. The case becomes easier to resolve if we interpret the issue as one of whether the counselor should give Helen the choice of receiving the information.

Legal cases about entitlement to information usually arise when a person is requesting that information. Here, Helen is not asking for information. It seems odd to ask whether she is "entitled" to have information thrust upon her because it is relevant to her health. Even when patients ask for information about themselves, the law usually considers the reasons the person seeks the information and the dangers involved in providing the information, rather than simply assuming that the patient is entitled to all information about him- or herself (*Gotkin v. Miller*). The law aside, rather than asking whether Helen is entitled to the information, it is probably better to ask whether she is entitled to decide whether she wants to receive the information.

Helen does not know she is at risk; she does not know she has a choice to make. She should be told that studies aimed at diagnosing her daughter necessarily reveal information about her, and she should be counseled about the full range of information that could have been discovered. She should be contacted and given the choice of whether to be informed. Her situation is like that of Ann and Jack in Case 4, with the important difference that Helen has had no indication that she may be at risk.

To deny Helen that choice would involve an unjustified level of paternalism. If the possibility of relevant information about her life is not presented to Helen, Natalie, with the counselor's collusion, will be substituting her view of her mother's best interests for her mother's own view. That is unacceptable in the absence of evidence that Helen is incompetent or, perhaps, a professional judgment that she is too fragile to receive bad news. Natalie's own, unexplored, possible conflicts of interest only strengthen the argument against allowing her wishes to control.

If, on the other hand, the information is thrust upon Helen without giving her a choice, the counselor will be imposing his or her own view that knowledge is better than ignorance. That, too, is unacceptable in this case, especially given our information about people's reactions to learning that they carry the gene for HD (Bloch 1992; Huggins 1992; Wiggins et al. 1992) and the red flag Natalie has raised about her mother's psychological equilibrium. This conclusion is strengthened, as noted earlier, by the lack of a public health reason to disclose and the fact that Helen could not use the information to avoid a bad health outcome.

Helen should be given the opportunity to make an informed choice about whether to be informed about test results she has not requested.

The Brothers

The informed choice approach also works for Natalie's brothers. They, too, should be told that testing performed on their family members may provide additional information about their risk for HD and asked whether they want to be informed of new results. Given their prior refusals, it is not likely that they will want to be informed, but the choice should be theirs. Their situation resembles that of the children in Case 8, "Mr. H.": All are aware that they are at risk for HD, and all have declined testing.

Things will get sticky if one brother asks to be informed and the other asks not to be informed, or if one or both brothers seek information and Helen refuses it. On those facts, the case would become like Cases 1, "Paul and Michael"; 2, "Father and Son"; and 6, "Kirsten and David," involving conflicts between persons who want information and those who decline it, in situations in which disclosure to one necessarily entails disclosure to others. In those cases, we concluded that persons who seek information relevant to their own health ought not to be denied information because another individual, even a close relative, will be upset by it. Of course, to the extent feasible, the counselor should try to protect persons who prefer not to learn bad news, but one person's preference for living with uncertainty should not outweigh another person's desire for knowledge. In this case the counselor could accurately inform one brother about his risk status without offering any comment on a sibling's risk.

Case 10 Mary Ann

Mary Ann, a twenty-year-old woman, is a member of a large family with multiple cases of breast and ovarian cancer. She has been tested for the BRCA1 gene at a research center and found to have a mutation that confers an 87 percent lifetime risk of developing breast cancer. Mary Ann is presently cancer-free.

Mary Ann's mother, Evelyn, is also a patient of Mary Ann's gynecologist. Two of Evelyn's three sisters were diagnosed with breast cancer at the ages of forty and forty-two, and her mother died of ovarian cancer at age fifty-seven. Evelyn is forty-nine. She is not participating in regular screening for either breast or ovarian cancer.

The gynecologist discusses a plan for cancer screening with Mary Ann. When she mentions that Evelyn also must now be diligent about her screening, Mary Ann asks the gynecologist not to discuss her test results with Evelyn, stating, "Mother couldn't take it. She is emotionally unstable."

Should Evelyn be told Mary Ann's test results? Is the accuracy of Mary Ann's assessment of her mother relevant?

Hereditary breast cancer accounts for approximately 5 percent to 10 percent of all breast cancer (Lynch et al. 1984). Mutations in the BRCA1 gene are thought to be responsible for about 50 percent of all inherited breast cancer (Easton et al. 1993). The BRCA1 gene is a probable tumor suppressor gene located on chromosome 17 at band q21 (Hall et al. 1990). As with many other tumor suppressor genes, germline mutations of BRCA1 are postulated to be transmitted in an autosomal dominant pattern (Newman et al. 1988). Cloned in October 1994, the gene is extremely large with exons spread over approximately 100,000 base pairs of genomic DNA (Miki et al. 1994; Castilla et al. 1994). Initial reports describe a variety of mutations in different family pedigrees, indicating that testing for individual familial mutations will be laborious (Miki et al. 1994; Novak 1994). Thus, widespread clinical testing is currently not available.

Although the gene is highly penetrant, identification of BRCA1 gene carriers will not predict with certainty whether a woman will develop cancer. However, women with germline mutations of BRCA1 have an 87 percent risk of developing breast cancer by age eighty-five and as high as a fifty-nine percent risk of breast cancer by age fifty (Ford et al. 1994). The risk of ovarian cancer is estimated to be 29 percent by age fifty and 44 percent by age seventy (Ford et al. 1994). Counseling can educate women about the need for vigilant screening to help detect cancers early, should they develop. Usually, the earlier the cancer is detected, the more amenable it is to treatment and thus the higher the likelihood of survival.

In this case, Mary Ann, the proband, has tested positive for a mutation in the BRCA1 gene. From this information alone we know that she is highly motivated and has participated in testing for BRCA1 conducted in a research testing center, since widespread testing is presently unavailable. With the determination that she is a gene carrier, we know she is at an increased risk for breast and ovarian cancer and probably colon cancer as well. She must be educated about recommended screening procedures for early detection of cancer, including monthly breast self-examination, biannual breast examination by a physician, and annual (or biannual) mammogram. For ovarian cancer, recommended screening procedures consist of frequent pelvic exams by a physician, transvaginal ultrasound, and use of Doppler-flow imaging.

Germline mutations can be transmitted on either the maternal or paternal allele. Given her pedigree information, Mary Ann's gene was most likely inherited from Evelyn. However, Mary Ann's father's family history should not be ignored. Men who carry the BRCA1 mutation may be at an elevated risk for prostate and colon cancer (Ford et al. 1994).

Even apart from the new information about Mary Ann, it is clear that Evelyn has an elevated risk of developing breast or ovarian cancer. With one affected first-degree relative, she would have a risk of breast or ovarian cancer two to three times that of the general population whether or not she carried the BRCA1 gene. With two affected first-degree relatives who had disease onset before age fifty, she would be characterized as high risk with approximately a 40 percent to 50 percent chance of developing breast cancer by age eighty (Hoskins et al. 1995). If her mother's cancer is added to the equation, Evelyn would be considered high risk, with a 50 percent chance of inheriting a probable gene mutation of a breast/ovarian cancer gene.

As discussed in earlier cases, predictive testing in Huntington disease (HD) has revealed that potential negative psychological consequences of testing for both the consultand and family members must be addressed. Lerman et al. (l994) surveyed 121 first-degree relatives (FDRs) of ovarian cancer patients for interest in and expectations about a potential genetic test for breast and ovarian cancer. Overall, 75 percent of those surveyed said they would want to be tested for BRCA1, and 20 percent said that they probably would want testing. Interest was positively associated with education, perceived likelihood of being a gene carrier, perceived risk of ovarian cancer, ovarian cancer worries, and mood disturbance. Significantly, 80 percent of FDRs expected to be very depressed when informed of a positive test result, 77 percent expected to be anxious, and 32 percent predicted an impairment in quality of life. One subject said she would consider suicide.

After receiving a positive test result, Mary Ann may be in a state of shock, anxiety, and perhaps depression. Her request to keep the news from her mother may be prompted by a desire to spare Evelyn the same anxiety and possible guilt. It is important for the physician to acknowledge the request as protective yet educate Mary Ann about the revised risks that may now confront her mother. This discussion need not occur at the same session as disclosure of test results, but could be addressed at another visit either by the physician or by the genetic counselor. Furthermore, the issue of disclosure of "family" information should have been discussed with Mary Ann during pretest counseling so that she could have anticipated this predicament.

Like Cases 7, "Robert," and 9, "Natalie," this case raises the issue of whether to adhere to a patient's request for confidentiality or warn a family member. Should the physician override Mary Ann's wishes and inform Evelyn of her revised risk?

In other cases, we have argued that it is important for persons to know that they are at risk, even if informing them conflicts with the request of another family member. A parallel case is health care providers' obligation to educate their patients about the potential health risks such as the relationship between smoking and cancer. If the patient is informed and subsequently refuses intervention to prevent or modify the health risk, and the health risk is not potentially harmful to others (unlike the situation in Case 11, "Maurice"), then the health care provider has discharged his or her responsibility.

As stated earlier, Evelyn's pedigree contains multiple cases of cancer. Perhaps Mary Ann's request is based on behavior or a verbal admission by Evelyn indicating that she anticipates the development of cancer and believes that screening is futile. Anxiety and cancer worries have been associated with lower rates of screening mammograms as well as reduction in the performance of breast self-examination. In the study by Lerman et al. (1994), 82 percent of FDRs felt they would be more in control of their lives with a positive test compared to 99 percent of those who received a negative test result. Evelyn's behavior may well reflect recognition of the magnitude of her risk. If her behavior reveals fatalism, then she is not unsuspecting, but is she informed? The gynecologist should explore with Evelyn her perception of her own cancer risk. She must be informed of the general population risk of cancer for her age, compared to her increased risk based on her family pedigree. Mary Ann's test results need not be disclosed in order to inform her, as Evelyn's risk is already known to be elevated beyond that of the general population.

In the case of cancer, unlike HD, it is important to know one's gene status or "potential for disease" based on family history, because the disease outcome can be modified. Does the gene test change Evelyn's perceived degree of cancer risk sufficiently to try to persuade Mary Ann to disclose her test results, or even to inform Evelyn of those results over Mary Ann's objections? We cannot predict Evelyn's response to being told she has a risk of developing cancer of 50 percent (based on her pedigree) or 87 percent (based on Mary Ann's genetic test). Predicting her response is difficult. Her behavior might suggest that she believes she has a 100 percent risk for disease; if so, informing her of any figure less than 100 percent may be good news and might actually encourage her to be screened. On the other hand, if she is given a 50 percent risk of disease and is still not motivated to begin screening measures, it is hard to see that a change in the odds will have an effect.

Evelyn's gynecologist's primary goal is to engage Evelyn in medical screening. When professionals give advice, they often do not explain every step of their thought processes, but clearly the doctor's information is given with the intention of benefiting Evelyn. Knowing what she already knows and what can be inferred from pedigree studies, if Evelyn is still not motivated, little will be gained by disclosing Mary Ann's test results. Evelyn should be warned of the gravity of her risk but without revealing Mary Ann's test results.

Case 11 *Maurice*

Maurice, a thirty-year-old man at risk for HD, is employed as a commercial airline pilot. He has told no one at work about his risk. After a relative went through presymptomatic testing, Maurice decided to pursue testing for himself. During pretest counseling, the counselor thoroughly explored issues of job performance and safety with Maurice. Given the expected age of onset in his family, the counselor stressed that if Maurice were to test positive, he had only a remote chance of being able to continue as an airline pilot long enough to reach the retirement age of forty-five and that he should think about alternatives. The counselor also stated that, considering the nature of his job, she hoped that Maurice would return for yearly neurological examinations in addition to undergoing the physicals required by the Federal Aviation Administration (FAA). He agreed to this arrangement.

The test results indicate that Maurice carries the gene for HD. When he learns this result, he states that he has no plans to tell anyone at work or to request a transfer to a supervisory position that pays more but has less prestige.

The counselor is troubled by this situation, given the implications for public safety. She is aware of the Tarasoff *ruling but is uncertain how it would apply to this situation. She seeks advice from several of her colleagues as well as lawyers, counselors, and ethicists. While the advice is somewhat contradictory, the majority of her consultants believes that she has a duty to inform the FAA of Maurice's risk if he refuses to do so.*

When Maurice returns for followup, the counselor questions him further about his plans for employment. He has made no specific plans; he says that he will continue to work as long as possible in his well-paid job. The counselor informs Maurice that she is troubled by the situation and reports the advice of her colleagues. Maurice becomes quite angry and upset. The counselor suggests that for everyone's protection, Maurice should have a baseline neuropsychological assessment and annual neurological examinations. The counselor tells Maurice that if abnormalities were found in either of these assessments, she would feel some pressure to disclose his genetic status to his employer, if he continues to refuse to do so. He declines to participate in this testing. He states that he does not want to give the counselor any information that might convince her that she needs to inform his employer.

The first question concerns the counselor's ethical and moral obligations. How should she balance the important yet mutually contradictory obligations of the patient's right to confidentiality versus the public's interest in safety?

Controversy surrounds the question of whether a duty exists to disclose to third parties information obtained in a genetic counseling session. The President's Commission (1983), acknowledging the difficulty of the issue, gave a set of necessary and sufficient conditions for overriding the duty to protect patient confidentiality and disclosing *to spouses or other at-risk family members.*

> A professional's ethical duty of confidentiality to an immediate patient or client can be overridden only if several conditions are satisfied: 1) Reasonable efforts to elicit voluntary consent to disclosure have failed; 2) there is a high probability both that harm will occur if the information is withheld and that the disclosed information will actually be used to prevent the harm; 3) the harm that identifiable individuals would suffer would be serious; and 4) appropriate precautions are taken to insure that only the genetic information needed for diagnosis and/or the treatment of the disease in question is disclosed. (44)

Unrelated third parties and employers were a different matter, however; the Commission argued that no results should be provided to insurers or employers without the explicit consent of the person screened (42).

The most relevant legal precedent is *Tarasoff v. University of California Board of Regents,* which asserted the duty of a therapist or mental health professional to warn against the violent actions of patients. Subsequent California cases have expressly limited the scope of the *Tarasoff* duty to circumstances involving a specifically identified or identifiable victim.

A number of other states have limited liability to cases where the patient has communicated a credible threat of violence against identified or identifiable persons. Some state courts have enlarged the scope of responsibility and adopted a broader theory of liability. These cases expand a therapist's liability beyond injuries to the identified or identifiable victim to include injuries to "reasonably foreseeable" victims of a patient whom the therapist knows or reasonably should have known was dangerous. Still other courts have concluded that a therapist's liability is not limited to identifiable victims, but extends to the class of persons whom the therapist could have reasonably foreseen as subject to an unreasonable risk of harm from the violence of a patient known to the therapist (Green and Barden 1992). At the very least, the counselor has a clear duty to act in a "reasonable (nonnegligent) manner." However, what is reasonable cannot be defined in advance with any certainty; it is likely to be determined by the court after the feared event has already occurred.

Thus, although the precedents suggest that a counselor may have a legal duty to disclose in some circumstances, including this one, they do not resolve the *moral* issue in this case. The law requires "reasonableness"—the meaning of which is a judgment call—and law and morality are not always congruent.

The general lines of a moral argument for disclosure to the employer are obvious. An airline pilot experiencing early symptoms of HD may make a mistake on the ground or in the air that costs the lives of many innocent people. The danger may be classified as serious. It is exacerbated by the fact that the first symptoms of HD may be subtle, and that they are unlikely to be picked up by routine physical examinations. To avoid legal liability in such a situation, at least one testing center has refused to test unless the prospective consultand first signs a form allowing disclosure of a positive result to an employer.

In fact, although these facts are sensational, the safety issue raised by this case is not as rare as might be supposed. Persons with HD play many roles that affect the safety of others; most, for example, drive automobiles, which suggests the issues of line drawing that this case raises.

Some of us feel that the counselor, at least in this extreme case, should insist on immediate disclosure to the employer, threatening to make the disclosure herself, if necessary. The majority resist this conclusion. They insist that in predictive testing, a distinction must be made between *current* and *future* danger. A truly presymptomatic individual carrying the HD gene (i.e., an individual who has a normal neurological examination, no psychiatric abnormalities, and no cognitive difficulties) has the same probability of having an accident as anyone who does not carry the HD gene. (One might argue that knowing that one carries the gene is disruptive and distracting in some way, but we have no data to support that, and all persons come to their work encumbered by distractions from other dimensions of their lives.) Thus, a presymptomatic person in a responsible position is not a present threat to public safety but *a potential threat at some unspecified time in the future.*

The existence of definite but future risk makes this case difficult. While reasonable persons might agree on a need to disclose eventually, deciding when to disclose raises serious questions that are not addressed by hastily coercing the patient.

For example, one must consider the long-term ramifications. A decision to inform might actually undermine the very thing the counselor is striving to protect, i.e., public safety. One argument for confidentiality is that it helps to provide a safe haven to which individuals seeking testing can turn in complete trust. When confidentiality is maintained, individuals who wish to behave responsibly can be tested and can use information about their genetic status to make intelligent, informed decisions. Suppose it becomes known that counselors will inform the employers of some persons who have tested positive. Persons who consider testing will confront a choice between ignorance of their genetic status and premature unemployment. Understandably, some will choose not to be tested and will work longer than is wise. Thus, from one point of view, standing for confidentiality amounts to a bet that the public is less at risk when people feel secure in the good faith of testing programs.

Furthermore, we cannot be sure that employers will understand genetic information or use it fairly. Previous experience with genetic screening programs has shown that a lack of knowledge concerning genetics can lead to oversimplified and unnecessary regulations. It is difficult for many people to comprehend the fact that predictive or presymptomatic testing can determine whether a person carries a gene for a particular disease, and yet tells *nothing* about the individual's current health status. If knowledgeable genetics professionals begin to warn employers of potentially dangerous employees, it is likely that the distinction between being symptomatic and being a gene carrier will become blurred, and consultands will suffer from misinformed bias. Counselors should feel an obligation to prevent consultands from being unjustly disadvantaged as a result of others' ignorance or incomplete information.

The issue of patient/consultand confidentiality cannot be taken lightly. Information about one's genetic risks is very personal, closely tied to one's identity or sense of self. The confidentiality promise counts for naught if it cannot be honored in cases like this one. The counselor knows that the consultand is not currently symptomatic. He is already subject to regular examinations by an FAA-approved physician, who is responsible for clearing him for work. Although the counselor may have some obligation to work with Maurice over time, and perhaps to try to persuade him to agree to have regular neurological examinations, it is better to reach this result by appealing to his sense of responsibility, rather than by a threat of disclosure.

Although the counselor will protect his confidentiality, Maurice himself has significant obligations in this situation. In the performance of his job-related duties, he is responsible for the lives of hundreds of passengers and others. He has a reasonable duty to act responsibly to ensure the welfare of innocent third parties, specifically a moral obligation to ensure the safety of his passengers. What does this obligation entail? Maurice's neurological examination at the time of testing was normal, indicating that he has not begun to show symptoms of HD. Assuming that is the case, Maurice does not pose any present danger to passengers.

Furthermore, if he were to inform his employer, he would run the risk of being dismissed from his job. It has not been entirely clear whether the Americans with Disabilities Act (ADA) protects individuals who are "presymptomatic." The definition of disability in the ADA includes being perceived to have a disability. Presymptomatic individuals suffering from discrimination (i.e., job loss) may be regarded as having a genetic condition that is potentially disabling and, therefore, would be covered (Alper 1995). On March 14, 1995, the Compliance Manual of the Equal Employment Opportunity Commission concluded that individuals who are subjected to discrimination on the basis of "genetic information related to illness, disease, or other disorder" are regarded as having disabling impairments (quoted in Alper 1995, p. 168). Ultimately, the question of whether the ADA covers presymptomatic individuals will be resolved in the courts.

In any case, Maurice confronts a real risk of losing his job. One might argue that in the absence of symptoms, he has no present obligation to inform his employers. However, a positive test means that eventually Maurice will develop symptoms. He has a clear obligation to avoid posing unreasonable risks to others. Although Maurice is required to have regular physical examinations as a condition of continued employment, the subtle early symptoms of HD are easily missed in clinical examination. It seems likely that his employer would require Maurice to undergo a more rigorous examination by a neurologist familiar with HD and its early manifestations, if his employer knew that he carried the gene for HD. Thus, if he does not inform his employer of his test result, he has an obligation to initiate well-informed and rigorous yearly physical examinations and assessments at his own initiative and expense. If and when he is found to be showing symptoms, he must inform his employer. At that point, Maurice would be considered disabled and would probably be covered under the ADA.

In sum: The remote possibility of a major air disaster in the future does not justify violating this man's confidentiality now. The situation is better handled by encouraging the consultand to have regular examinations and by helping him to work as long as he can safely and effectively continue.

If Maurice becomes symptomatic, however, the situation changes. Then the threat of danger is current and escalating. At that point the counselor should try to convince Maurice to disclose his illness to his employer. If he refuses, informing his employer without his permission is morally acceptable and in keeping with the counselor's moral obligation to protect innocent third parties.

Indeed, if Maurice refuses to establish a program of future examinations or assessments, he abdicates his moral responsibility to protect the safety of his passengers. In that situation, the counselor may well feel complicit in arrangements that put others at serious risk. She would be entirely justified in sharing her discomfort in this situation with Maurice and insisting that he agree to schedule a series of regular neurological examinations that she can monitor. They can negotiate an arrangement with which they are comfortable. Should he refuse to cooperate, however, informing his employer may be acceptable, even mandatory.

Case 12 Mr. L.

Mr. L., a twenty-seven-year-old man, has applied for a $250,000 life insurance policy. His mother recently died of Huntington disease. In its family history section, the insurance company's form specifically asks about mental illness or suicide. The form also includes space for information on the age of parents and siblings, if living, or, if deceased, for their cause of death and age at death. Mr. L. is worried: If the insurance company learns that he is at risk of carrying the gene for HD, it may ask him to undergo presymptomatic testing, refuse to issue a policy to him, or charge him higher premiums. Although he has begun counseling for presymptomatic testing for HD, Mr. L. has not decided whether to be tested. How should the counselor advise him? Would the counselor be justified in helping Mr. L. attempt to beat the insurance system?

Mr. L's fears are not unfounded. The literature on genetics issues in insurance has tended to focus on health insurance; less has been written about life insurance. Similarities and contrasts are apparent. For example, both health and life insurers may subject applicants to individual risk classification and medical underwriting to determine whom to cover and what to charge. This practice is less common in health insurance, which is often provided as a fringe benefit with employment, particularly if the employer has a large workforce. In fact, however, instances of genetic discrimination have been reported by applicants for both health and life insurance (Billings et al. 1992; Barash 1994; Geller et al. 1996). "Skimming" (accepting only the applicants who have the lowest risks) is not unknown among life insurers.

To assess the risks of coverage and assign proportionate premiums, the industry must rely on the candor and honesty of applicants for insurance. The entire system is based on the principle of charging equal premiums for individuals who have equal expected risks of loss. That system works when both insurers and insureds are equally informed about all factors that bear on the assignment of an individual to an appropriate risk classification. The life insurance industry is highly sensitive to the problem of adverse selection, the tendency of individuals who know they are at higher risk to overpurchase insurance compared to the rest of the population. This tendency may threaten the industry if insureds have information about their health status that is unavailable to insurers. From the industry's point of view, insureds who conceal information undermine the system.

Concealment is difficult, because insurance companies require applicants to sign waivers of confidentiality, which open their medical records for inspection. Insurers may gain access to underwriting information by obtaining medical histories or medical records, by requiring statements from physicians, or by asking applicants to undergo medical tests stipulated by the company (Nelkin and Tancredi 1989). If an insurance company is one of 700 members of the Medical Information Bureau (MIB), a central clearinghouse for data on applicants, it can obtain additional information. MIB members pool data on potential insureds, and one company's adverse decision may effectively preclude an applicant from obtaining coverage from others.

Deliberately withholding or falsifying information on an insurance application may constitute fraud. Many state laws contain contestability limits. For example, Indiana law allows claims to be contested on a life insurance policy within two years and on a health insurance policy within three years after issuance (Indiana Code Annotated). After the period specified by statute, applicants' misstatements cannot be used to void a health insurance policy *"except fraudulent misstatements"* (Preheim, March 31, 1994; emphasis added).

Well-established practice has created a climate of public acceptance for disclosure of confidential information to insurers. This stress on disclosure may challenge patients' legitimate expectations of confidentiality and create conflicts of interest for health care providers.

The specific problem we confront is whether disclosure of genetic information is comparable to disclosure of other kinds of medically relevant information. Although the insurance industry has stated that it is not requiring genetic testing, it is clear that insurers are likely to want access to genetic information. Many health insurers regard genetic testing as a threat to their companies' financial well-being, unless test results are available to underwriters; this attitude is likely to prevail among life insurers as well.

Some have proposed that genetic information and nongenetic information should be considered separately and treated differentially in terms of disclosure. Disorders due to one's genetic heritage are said to be less subject to one's voluntary control than disorders that have an environmental or behavioral component (Karjala 1992). Confidentiality of genetic information may constitute a special case because genetic disease affects entire families as well as individual patients, because it figures in sensitive decisions about reproduction, because of the history of misuse of genetic information, and because of fears of stigmatization and discrimination (NIH-DOE 1993). The possibility—or the likelihood—that insurers will fail to master the complexities of information derived from genetic tests and thus will use this information inappropriately in underwriting (NIH-DOE 1993) increases the danger that genetic information will exacerbate problems of access to insurance (Karjala 1992).

However, differentiating genetic from nongenetic information may not be practical or possible, due to the difficulty of distinguishing genetic factors from environmental factors in the etiology of diseases such as cancer and the difficulty of categorizing health risks as purely genetic or nongenetic. It is problematical to suggest that insurers' decisions should be based on the degree to which illness is under the patient's control. Moreover, it is impractical to expect physicians to exclude genetic information from medical records that are routinely sent in their entirety at insurers' request.

With this background in mind, we return to the case of Mr. L. If he is not a resident of a state that bans such practices, the insurance company is free to ask him to undergo testing for HD, deny coverage outright, or assign higher premiums. Mr. L. has not sought genetic testing, for whatever reasons. In various studies, persons at risk have identified a variety of factors that discourage testing, including the possible loss of health insurance (Quaid and Morris 1993).

Requiring applicants for insurance to undergo presymptomatic testing as a condition of coverage has the effect of discouraging individuals at risk of HD from participation in the insurance pool. Whether or not this practice amounts to genetic discrimination under the Americans with Disabilities Act, insurers' underwriting policies encourage those at risk to conceal information from their health care providers for fear of disclosure to third parties, jeopardizing the indispensable candor of the professional-patient relationship.

In terms of insurance coverage, genetic counselors find themselves working amidst social policies that offer no unambiguous options. Genetic counselors have an obligation to advise consultands of the adverse effects of presymptomatic testing, including the possible loss of insurability. Persons considering testing should be fully apprised of all relevant risks.

Some counselors apparently go further, however. Anecdotal evidence indicates that they may advise patients to apply for life or disability insurance *before* undergoing presymptomatic testing for HD, while their genetic status is still unknown. Counselors may also advise consultands to exercise caution in responding to insurers' application forms, limiting their answers to the specific information requested. For example, if a parent died of pneumonia secondary to Huntington disease, the consultand might describe the cause of death as pneumonia and refrain from volunteering the information that the parent had been diagnosed with HD.

Some critics regard this approach as morally problematic. They point out that while counselors may argue that their advice is based on their wish to promote consultands' best interests, lack of candor or outright deception on the part of the consultand may injure others: If the risk of HD is not fully disclosed by some insureds, other policyholders' premiums may be unfairly increased. Thus, failure to mention HD in that context seems to default on the consultands' duties to others. On the other hand, one can argue that neither counselor nor consultand has any duty to *volunteer* more information than that requested, especially if the context is one in which basic human needs are involved.

Thus, some may feel that counselors are more justified in helping consultands to beat the system in the case of health insurance than life insurance. Health care has been described as an "opportunity good" that enables other goods, one to which all members of society are entitled (Karjala 1992). Because the United States lacks a nationalized system of health care provision, access to health care for many depends on the availability of private insurance. Some argue that for counselors to offer consultands advice on gaming this system seems a matter of simple justice, perhaps a kind of conscientious objection. Even if there is such an argument, however, it does not apply to life insurance.

Life insurance, while important, is arguably a less urgent need.[2] In Mr. L's case, it is appropriate for the counselor to disclose the risks associated with testing, but assisting him to obtain insurance coverage through fraud or deception goes too far. While counselors are consultand advocates, that is not all they are: They are not exempt from general duties of truthfulness and public accountability.

---

2. Some have proposed that minimal life insurance should be made available to all. Important issues raised by such a proposal must be addressed, including the definition of minimal coverage, whether underwriting is appropriate and at what level, and how such a program would be funded (NIH-DOE 1993; Karjala 1992).

Case 13 Mr. Crawford

Mr. Crawford's son married a woman at risk for HD. The couple, now divorced, were married for eight years and had a son and a daughter. The boy is now eight years old, and the girl is six. These children are at 25 percent risk for HD. Mr. Crawford believes that the mother of his former daughter-in-law has been diagnosed with HD; the former daughter-in-law has repeatedly said that she is not interested in testing for herself. Mr. Crawford has other children and grandchildren; a widower of significant means, he has been diagnosed with inoperable cancer. He wishes to treat his grandchildren equitably, but he believes that special needs require special commitments. He contemplates setting up a trust fund for his son's children to ensure adequate care for them if they should develop HD. In order to know whether he should make these arrangements, Mr. Crawford wants to have his grandchildren tested.

This case raises two significant issues. The first is whether health professionals should test children for the presence of the HD mutation, assuming that an appropriate proxy so requests; the second is decision making for children when the family is divided.

Should the Children Be Tested?

The first issue—whether children should ever be tested for HD— can be focused narrowly or broadly. Most of the written commentary on the narrow issue takes the view that children should not be tested for late-onset diseases (HDSA 1989, 1994; Harper and Clarke 1990; Harper 1992; Quaid 1993, Quaid 1994). Sharpe (1993, 1994) has challenged this view, basing his argument on the broader principle of family autonomy. Sharpe's argument is strengthened if we note that the consent of one parent generally provides sufficient legal justification for performance of a medical procedure on a child. If this legal doctrine offers a tight analogy, it will suggest that children should be tested for HD at their parents' request. (See Wertz et al. 1994.)

A minority of our group holds that the disanalogies are not strong enough to force us to depart from this rule. They argue that young children are not able to exercise their autonomy rights; as a society, we have authorized parents to exercise those rights for their children for several reasons: The parents know more than the children; all things being equal, parents can be counted on to care more about the children than anybody else; some prerogatives should accompany the parents' duties toward their children. The family represents the unit in which the child's values and sense of self will be formed. Thus, we should depart from the rule of parental control only when there is real reason to doubt the parents' capacity or concern for the child, when circumstances clearly reveal that their interest conflicts with that of the child, or when obvious public health considerations exist. None of those exceptions is relevant in this case.

These arguments in favor of parental prerogatives are supported by two further considerations. First is the claim that testing does not necessarily imply that the child will be informed of the results. Parents often know things that they do not immediately share with their children. Results of an HD test could be kept from the children, perhaps indefinitely. Second, the risks the children would incur as a result of testing are highly speculative. Testing may reveal that they do not carry the mutation, relieving a major source of anxiety. Even if one or both of the children are found to be HD gene carriers—and even if the children are informed of their status—it is not certain that this knowledge will lead to worse consequences for the children than unawareness or uncertainty. Informed parents may stigmatize or overprotect the children, but these outcomes should not be assumed. Both testing and not testing involve risks to the child (Sharpe 1993, 1994). Generally, we overrule parental refusal of treatment only in a few cases in which it is certain that the treatment will benefit the child. What reason is there to believe the children are more likely to be injured by testing than by refusing to test?

Strong as these arguments are, our majority feels that the children should not be tested for HD, even if testing is requested by one or both parents. Our argument hinges on some distinctive features of HD at this juncture in the development of diagnosis and treatment. HD is a late-onset disease of high penetrance for which no known cure or treatment is available. Development of symptoms before the age of thirty is possible but unusual. Thus, it is extremely difficult to see how testing can be understood to be in the children's medical interest. If the children carry the gene, absolutely nothing can be done medically. In contrast to other genetic diseases (including FAP and ADPKD, which appear in other cases), nothing is lost medically by waiting and allowing the children to decide for themselves whether they want to be tested. The sole and certain effects of testing now are in the minds of persons who are informed of the results of the test. The possibility of a conflict of interest between parents and children cannot be ruled out.

Given these medical facts, testing must be justified by either the social interest of the children, or the interest of someone else—characteristically other member(s) of the family. In this case, the best argument for the test is benefit for the children. If we take Mr. Crawford's claims at face value, he lovingly wants to give them the best possible safety net. However, other pathologies or trauma may shorten or impair the children's lives. Thus, even on his own terms, the special benefit Mr. Crawford means to base on test results is highly speculative. We must consider the possibility that Mr. Crawford's real intention is to favor the other children in the distribution of his estate, avoiding a "bad investment" in a child who carries the HD mutation. (See the discussion of "preselection" in Case 15, "Jimmy.")

Moreover, children have real interests beyond material security, and it is obvious that parental authority cannot be unlimited. The real question is whether the state or health professionals may override parental choice and, if so, what goods for the child will justify such an override. Many of these goods are appropriate matters of parental preference, bias, or tradition, e.g., religious training, but not all; parents should be prevented from making choices that put their children at great risk, and the act of testing the child for HD is both risky and irrevocable.

Preservation of bodily integrity is not the only valid reason for resisting parental choice. Another is preserving a viable self-image and basis for self-respect in the child. To be sure, knowledgeable persons will differ in good faith over the necessary psychosocial preconditions for development of self-respect, but they also differ about the necessities of bodily integrity. It is clear that many adults at risk for HD do not seek presymptomatic testing; they prefer not to resolve the issue of their own risk (Evers-Kiebooms et al. 1989; Quaid and Morris 1993). The literature contains reports of negative consequences even when the test shows that the proband is not at risk (Huggins et al. 1992). It is obvious that this information is emotionally supercharged. In these circumstances, it seems more prudent to defer securing it until children have developed to the point where they, ideally supported by their families, may decide to request it for themselves. We repeat: It is the decision to be tested that is irrevocable.

What Do the Parents Want?

The facts of the case do not make clear whether the children's parents favor or oppose the tests. If the parents oppose testing, we agree that the children should not be tested. The grandfather's responsibilities for the children and any rights of proxy he may have are of less weight than those of the children's parents.

The case is more difficult, however, if the divorced parents disagree. A plausible situation would be that the mother, who is at risk, opposes testing, and the father, eager to protect his children from any eventuality, favors testing. The divorce proceeding may have awarded custody rights to one of the parents, with the power to make major health care decisions; this disposition may settle the issue as a matter of law. However, the decree may award shared decision-making power to the parents. We are not clear as to how to resolve this dispute on the moral level, and in any case it is moot for the majority.

A side issue in this case arises from the fact that a positive test on one of the children would reveal that their mother carries the HD mutation. Although she has said that she does not wish to be tested, given our resolution of other cases (e.g., Cases 1, "Paul and Michael," and 2, "Father and Son"), we cannot base a refusal to test the children on her wishes. We oppose testing Mr. Crawford's grandchildren but for their own sake, not primarily out of consideration for their mother.

Case 14 Mr. and Mrs. Anderson

A genetic counselor receives a call from Mr. and Mrs. Anderson, who are foster parents. They have been caring for a two-year-old girl almost from her birth, and they want to adopt her. The child's mother has been diagnosed with HD with an onset in the early to mid-twenties. Mr. and Mrs. Anderson want to have the child tested to see whether she carries the HD gene. If she does not carry the gene, they will proceed with the adoption. If she is a gene carrier, the adoption agency has alluded to a fund that will be set up to care for her, since it appears obvious to them that no other couple will want to adopt her. When the clinic informed Mr. and Mrs. Anderson that its policy is not to test children, the couple contacted a lawyer. The lawyer approached the counselor and stated that she is obliged to do what is in the child's best interest. The lawyer claims that is to test the child.

We laid out some of the issues involved in presymptomatic testing of children in another case (Case 13, "Mr. Crawford"). In that case, our majority felt that potential risks outweighed the potential benefits of testing children. We argued that conjectural nonmedical benefits were insufficient to override concern about family stigmatization and psychological risks. In effect, we established a prima facie presumption against testing children for the HD mutation.

This case escalates the stakes considerably for the child. Testing does not offer medical benefits, but we subscribe to the conventional view that it is better to grow up in a loving home than in an institution or as a ward of the state.

A minority disagreed with our conclusion in Case 13, "Mr. Crawford," and here their arguments are consistent. They argue that a negative test presents no problem. If the test is positive, the Andersons can relinquish the child, and the adoption agency can withhold the information from her until she becomes psychologically mature, sexually active, or whatever the appropriate time seems to be. In other words, there is a 50 percent chance of a happy outcome from the test. On the other hand, if the child tests positive for the gene, she need not be informed of the test result.

Other factors may strengthen this argument. All persons learn about their fate as children: They may learn about the unattractive features or physique they have inherited, about the limits of their natural talents and/or those of their parents, about constrained financial resources. Fate comes in many forms. We do not assume that children should not have this kind of information; we define a good home as one that makes them feel loved and able to cope with reality. We believe that parents should help children grow in the face of adversity; we do not believe that they should help their children to pretend that adversity does not exist or support them in an attitude of denial. Do we want to make an exception to these considerations in the case of a genetic disease? How does such a case differ?

It is certainly not unreasonable for prospective adoptive parents to want to know whether the child they may adopt carries a gene for a serious genetic disease, even if onset is likely to occur after the child leaves home. They may make a cool calculation of their resource budget to maximize their financial and emotional investment; they may want to engage in emotional protection, avoiding worry and heartache. One might argue that it would be preferable for them to rise above these feelings and attitudes, but they can hardly be characterized as unreasonable or irrational, and their request can scarcely be dismissed out of hand.

Nevertheless, a majority of our group feels that the child should not be tested. Our arguments are as follows. First, this request comes from foster parents who have no special standing with respect to this child at the moment. They are not the parents; they want the test in order to decide if they are willing to become parents. While the Andersons' interest in the information is entirely understandable and reasonable, it does not follow that testing to relieve their uncertainty is in the child's interest.

Second, while the child has a 50 percent chance of a substantial benefit—adoption into this family—she also has a 50 percent risk of a substantial loss. It will be much more difficult to place a known mutation carrier than a child whose genotype is uncertain. That is not to say that no foster or adoptive parents will appear for a child known to carry the HD mutation: We have anecdotal evidence to the contrary. If the child is not tested, the adoption agency can honestly report uncertainty; that possibility is lost once the test is done, for the agency will then have a legal duty to report any information available, if asked (Preheim, March 22, 1994).

Third, it is of some relevance that the majority of young adults who know themselves to be at risk for HD do not opt for testing (Morris et al. 1988). These data are based on limited samples; they do not establish general probabilities, let alone moral certitude, but they should give us pause. Should we seek to acquire knowledge about someone that many individuals in a similar situation do not seek to know about themselves?

Again, the specifics of HD are of the greatest relevance to our reasoning. If the test offered the possibility of medical benefit, we might reach a different conclusion. (See Cases 15, "Jimmy," and 16, "Harriet," for example.)

Two general considerations strengthen our position. Exactly how much adoptive parents should be told about the child they contemplate adopting is a difficult issue. We agree that they should be informed of factors that bear on the child's health while the child is in their home. Is it clear that they should have been told that this child was at risk for HD—a late-onset disorder? While it seems strange to give them that information without being willing to confirm the diagnosis, it may be worse to set a precedent for genetic testing of prospective adoptees. As genetic knowledge increases, few children will pass those tests with flying colors. In our case, the Andersons should be told that the child is at risk for HD, and the rationale for refusing to test should be explained to them.

Of course, this conclusion about testing children before adoption assumes a general social policy of not testing children. If parents can have their legal children (biological or adopted) tested, then the clinic's refusal to test merely sets up a scenario in which the prospective parents adopt, then test, then either return the child as damaged goods or find themselves in the position of the parents discussed in Case 13, "Mr. Crawford."

Legally, it does not seem to be the case that adoption agencies have a duty to perform genetic tests on children. The closest precedent to the contrary seems to be an Illinois statue that requires that children who are in the custody of the Children and Family Services Department be tested for human immunodeficiency virus at the request of the adoptive parents (Preheim, March 22, 1994). This law seems to be the exception that proves the rule, and so called wrongful adoption torts are "premised on active misrepresentation and not passive nondisclosure, let alone failure to investigate genetic information" (Preheim, March 22, 1994, 8).

Finally, the strongest argument against our conclusion may be that it may discourage the practice of adoption. We do not advocate a policy of complete nondisclosure of medical or genetic risks to adoptive parents. We cannot keep adoption policies from becoming a kind of triage in which children perceived to be the least risky are taken first. However, we can refuse to acquire information that is likely to damage the child psychologically or socially, that enables no enhanced medical care, and that is irrelevant to the decisions of a loving family during a child's formative years.

Case 15 Jimmy

Mrs. Brown, who has been on dialysis for five years due to autosomal dominant polycystic kidney disease, requests genetic testing for her fifteen-year-old son, Jimmy, who wants to play football and participate in other contact sports. Although a recent ultrasound examination of Jimmy showed no cysts, Mrs. Brown is adamant that she sees signs similar to her own as a youngster. She is convinced that Jimmy, unlike her two other children, carries the gene for ADPKD and will soon develop problems.

A psychological examination, recommended by the school because of failing grades and behavior problems, indicates that Jimmy is suffering from depression and anxiety.

This case differs from our other cases involving the testing of children (Cases 13, "Mr. Crawford," and 14, "Mr. and Mrs. Anderson") in two ways. First, the biological parent of a minor is requesting testing, and second, testing for ADPKD has implications for treatment.

ADPKD occurs at a frequency of 1 to 5 per 1,000 live births and is characterized by the early onset of renal hypertension and failure. Each child of an affected parent has a 50 percent chance of inheriting the gene that causes the disease. Clinical onset of this disorder typically occurs in the third to fifth decade of life, although cases of early onset have been reported (Michaud et al. 1994). For unknown reasons, the age at which symptoms begin varies both within and between families. This variability is important because onset determines the need for medical treatment, dietary therapy, dialysis, and renal transplant. The standard procedure is to monitor individuals at risk with ultrasound to check for the presence of renal cysts. Ultrasound detection is quite effective in diagnosing ADPKD before the onset of symptoms.

In 1985 Reeders et al. identified chromosome 16 as the site of at least one gene for ADPKD (PKD 1). This discovery enabled predictive testing using linkage. In 1988, Kimberling et al. suggested that not all cases of ADPKD were linked to the PKD 1 locus on chromosome 16. In 1993, Peters et al. assigned a second gene for ADPKD to chromosome 4.

However, it appears that more than 90 percent of families with ADPKD are linked to chromosome 16. In 1994, the gene for ADPKD was found on chromosome 16 (The European Polycystic Kidney Disease Consortium 1994) and direct genetic testing is now possible. To facilitate monitoring symptoms in those at highest risk, genetic testing is recommended (Caskey 1992). If Jimmy is to be tested, Mrs. Brown must first be tested to determine whether she has the mutation for ADPKD1. Once a mutation has been identified, Jimmy can be tested directly for the same mutation. Testing for ADPKD2 is not currently available.

Difficulty in determining Jimmy's best interests is compounded in this case by the phenomenon of the "preselection" of a minor in a family with a significant history of genetic disease. Preselection, a recognized phenomenon in the social psychology of families, refers to the singling out of an asymptomatic individual at risk and predicting that he or she will eventually become affected. Preselection is thought to fulfill several functions. First, it may serve as a means of containing the family's anxiety about the threat of the genetic disorder. A sense of freedom from the disease for the other siblings is purchased at the expense of the preselected individual. Second, preselection helps to organize a family's experience by assigning the roles of the healthy and the sick rather than leaving that to chance. Third, the preselected individual may function as a scapegoat for family problems that are unrelated to genetics (Kessler 1988).

Preselection may have a profound effect on an individual's functioning. Not uncommonly, a person who has been preselected to become ill may have major difficulties in choosing a life path. The preselected person may find it difficult to imagine a future that is already overshadowed by the threat of serious illness, or the family may direct resources and attention away from an individual who is thought to have fewer chances for a normal life. Preselection may also have serious psychological effects, including low self-esteem and periodic depression (Kessler 1988).

In this case, his mother has preselected fifteen-year-old Jimmy to develop ADPKD. The fact that a recent examination by ultrasound shows no evidence of renal cysts appears to have had no effect on Mrs. Brown's expectations despite the fact that ultrasound has been shown to be highly effective in monitoring the onset of disease in unaffected individuals. The case suggests that Jimmy's failing grades, behavior problems, and bouts of depression and anxiety may be due at least in part to preselection.

Despite these complications, if Jimmy's mother requests testing and Jimmy wants to be tested, there appears to be no reason not to test him. However, what if Jimmy does not want to be tested? Should testing proceed?

Generally, parents or guardians may consent to actions that will affect their children. However, although no general requirement of benefit to the child exists, and parental decisions are not monitored to ascertain whether they benefit the child, parents are not given carte blanche. Parental requests alone do not justify unnecessary treatment or withholding lifesaving treatment from a child. Children should not be considered possessions of their parents or mere means to the satisfaction of parental desires. Moreover, at fifteen, Jimmy has legitimate insight into his own interests. We see no justification for testing Jimmy against his will.

What if Jimmy wanted testing and his mother did not want him to be tested? In that case, we would need to look at exceptions to the general rule requiring parental consent. One exception is the "mature minor rule," usually applied to adolescents aged fifteen to eighteen, which allows physicians to proceed with the consent of a minor patient who has demonstrated sufficient maturity of understanding and intelligence. This rule is sometimes limited to fairly trivial medical procedures. Invoking it here would require some assessment of Jimmy's ability to comprehend the risks and benefits of the choice before him. If a determination could be made that Jimmy was sufficiently mature to act in his own best interest in this instance, it might be appropriate to proceed with testing without parental consent.

Jimmy may want testing; he may explicitly refuse it; or, as this case is written, Jimmy's desires regarding testing may be difficult to discern. In the absence of clarity regarding his wishes, the issue becomes whether to conduct testing that is not medically indicated at Mrs. Brown's request. At a minimum, several issues must be explored with her and with Jimmy before he is tested. Why is she requesting testing? What is it that she hopes to gain either for Jimmy or for herself? Is she requesting testing in order to confirm her own suspicions that he carries the mutation despite receiving a clean bill of health by ultrasound? If so, it seems legitimate to ask whether that is adequate reason to proceed. Might there be other considerations of which we are not aware?

What benefits are to be gained through testing in this case? The genetic testing of a person at risk for ADPKD, in contrast to HD, may offer medical benefits. Testing may be helpful as a means of increasing medical surveillance for those at highest risk. However, because Jimmy already appears to be following the recommendations for medical monitoring, it is unclear whether additional medical benefits could be obtained through testing.

Could testing provide psychological benefits? If testing indicates that Jimmy is not a gene carrier, one may assume that he will experience a great sense of relief, a definite benefit. On the other hand, his mother might be correct, and Jimmy may be found to be a gene carrier. An important point to consider in weighing the risks and benefits of testing is that Jimmy is already suffering from depression and anxiety. Although the case suggests that his psychological state stems from preselection, other factors may be relevant. For example, we have little information about the effect on the family of Mrs. Brown's illness and dialysis. Whatever the cause of his current difficulties, it is important that the counselor explore these issues with Jimmy prior to testing. If Jimmy is reacting to being considered a gene carrier despite the lack of objective evidence, his current psychological state is a major clue to the reaction he is likely to have if he is indeed found to be a carrier and suggests that great caution is in order.

Testing Jimmy against his will is wrong. Testing is acceptable if he and his mother clearly agree to request it. If his choice cannot be determined, a process of consultation should be undertaken. Jimmy should be tested only if it becomes clear that testing accords with his preference and serves his interest.

Case 16 Harriet

Harriet, a thirty-four-year-old woman with familial adenomatous poly-posis is referred by the gastrointestinal clinic. She has four children ages seven, nine, twelve, and sixteen. She is requesting that the children un-dergo direct gene testing to determine their FAP status. Genetic testing is also requested by the gastroenterologist, who would use the information to determine treatment approaches.

In our case discussions regarding the testing of children at risk for Hunt-ington disease, the majority opposed testing a child for a late-onset, non-preventable, nontreatable degenerative disorder. (See Cases 13, "Mr. Crawford," and 14, "Mr. and Mrs. Anderson.") FAP clearly represents a different scenario. Screening begins in childhood for a potential disease onset in childhood. Therefore, genetic testing of a child at risk for FAP can prevent morbidity and mortality. This benefit can be gained, how-ever, only with an accurate clinical diagnosis and mutational analysis of the affected individuals.

FAP is a well-defined familial cancer syndrome characterized by the presence of hundreds of polyps dispersed throughout the colon and rectum. Variant additional features may include polyps in the upper gastrointestinal tract, extraintestinal manifestations such as osteomas and epidermoid cysts, desmoid tumors, thyroid tumors, and congenital hypertrophy of the retinal pigment epithelium. FAP is inherited as an autosomal dominant condition with high penetrance (greater than 90 percent). Offspring of an affected individual are at 50 percent risk of in-heriting the disorder. Clinical manifestations, including multiple polyps, may be identifiable in childhood. Medical screening of potential gene car-riers, recommended to begin around age eleven, includes annual endos-copy of the colon and rectum. In those individuals in whom extensive polyposis is identified, prophylactic total colectomy is recommended due to the virtual certainty that they will develop colo-rectal cancer.

The gene responsible for FAP is located on chromosome 5 at q21 and is designated APC for adenomatous polyposis coli. Direct gene testing is available to detect familial mutations in the APC gene (Powell, Petersen, et al. 1992, Powell, Zilz, et al. 1992).

Prior to the availability of direct gene testing, counseling and clinical management were based on linkage results. For individuals designated as noncarriers of FAP, clinical follow-up consisted of a baseline flexible sigmoidoscope exam at age eleven and then every three years until age thirty-five. Those identified as gene positive continued annual endoscopy until polyps were found and were then counseled to consider prophylactic total colectomy. Recommendations have now been revised for those who test gene negative by direct mutational analysis of the APC gene. A baseline flexible sigmoidoscopy is still recommended at age eleven, but then again only at ages eighteen, twenty-five, and thirty-five. This regimen is designed to guard against false negative test results as well as possible tissue mosaicism or a de novo mutation.

General medical guidelines have been established for recommending the initiation of screening. However, these guidelines are sometimes modified in response to familial variations in disease onset. For example, if polyps begin to develop in childhood, screening may be recommended as early as age eight to ten. The appropriate age for genetic testing may then coincide with the timing of disease screening. In this case, a counselor may consider testing the seven- and nine-year-olds, if this family is characterized by early onset of disease. Otherwise, the counselor may suggest waiting until eleven years, the time usually recommended for the initiation of screening.

Among the issues to be addressed by the counselor, one would include the benefit of testing to Harriet and her children. One of the key recommendations from a recent report of the United Kingdom Clinical Genetics Society was that predictive genetic testing of children would be appropriate only if disease onset regularly occurred in childhood or if effective therapeutic interventions were available (Clinical Genetics Society [U.K.] 1994). Clearly, a case can be made for testing Harriet's twelve- and sixteen-year-old children. At these ages, medical screening normally would have begun. The screening is generally unpleasant, possibly embarrassing, and expensive. The child may need to follow a special endoscopy preparation diet prior to examination. This diet encourages liquids with the aim of cleaning out the colon. Enemas or suppositories are sometimes used. As stated earlier, it is recommended that individuals who are at risk or gene positive undergo annual endoscopy.

If either or both of these children test negative, screening can be reduced, sparing them the unpleasant examinations and loss of school time and possibly reducing the time off work for a parent who would accompany the child for screening. This outcome could also reduce health care expenses for both the family and the third party payer. A gene-positive test, on the other hand, would have the potential benefit of stressing the importance and determining the frequency of regular screening and may also allow time for adjustment to the eventual recommendation of a colectomy and ileostomy.

Suppose one of Harriet's two older children rejects testing. As long as medical screening is continued, the child's health will be protected. Should the child begin to develop polyps, genetic testing will be irrelevant. If not, screening will proceed annually until a decision is made to modify the timing. A more significant medical consequence would be for one child to refuse medical screening. This situation may be compared to the widely publicized story of Billy Best, who fled his Massachusetts home to resist chemotherapy for Hodgkin's disease. Although the law has allowed teenagers to receive medical treatment without parental permission in some situations, the law has not clarified teenagers' right to refuse treatment. The right to consent to medical care does not necessarily include the right to refuse care, because the consequences of consent and refusal may differ dramatically. This issue is legally unsettled.

Teenagers are appropriately involved in decision making about their health care. They can assent to medical screening or genetic testing. They also need the opportunity to be informed about the consequence of their decisions and possible options for care. The counselor and gastroenterologist can assist in providing education.

Testing for Harriet's younger children could wait until age eleven, unless the pedigree dictates otherwise. Because testing offers specific medical benefits despite the uncertain psychological consequences of testing children at age eleven, it would be difficult to argue against a parental request for testing at age seven or nine. The parents may be asked to consider postponing testing of the younger children to allow for the necessary interaction and attention to emotional and psychological reactions that will arise from disclosure of test results for the two older children. It might be helpful to include the gastroenterologist in the counseling process to discuss the medical implications of both a gene-positive and a gene-negative test result.

In summary, medical screening for FAP is clearly in the best interest of the child, and genetic testing may be in the best interest of the child. A gene-negative test will free the child and family from the risks, burdens, and costs of annual screening; a gene-positive test may reinforce compliance with medical screening and allow for acceptance of eventual surgery.

Case 17 Charley

At the urging of Charley's mother, a geneticist referred Charley, a six-year-old child, for testing for HD. A pediatric neurologist had diagnosed the child with Tourette's syndrome with some obsessive compulsive behavior. However, Liz, Charley's mother, claimed that his behavior was atypical and unpredictable, and she wanted to rule out HD. Charley's father has been diagnosed with HD; his symptoms appeared at about age twenty-six, and DNA analysis detected 51 and 18 CAG repeats. Liz reported that her exhusband's behavior was violent and abusive, and the couple has been divorced for approximately one year.

The HD testing protocol was discussed with Liz at length, as well as the issue of testing minors only under compelling medical circumstances. Should Charley be tested?

Our majority has opposed genetic testing for HD for minors because no treatment is available, no medical benefit accrues from presymptomatic diagnosis, and the risks of stigmatization and discrimination outweigh any nonmedical benefit that may derive from testing. The relatively small proportion of adults at risk who elect testing testifies to the profound impact of presymptomatic diagnosis.

Although some voices have been raised in dissent, the testing community appears to be reaching consensus that the decision to undergo testing should be made by informed adults. For example, HDSA guidelines originally recommended predictive testing only for persons at least 18 years of age. (HDSA 1989) Revised guidelines state:

> Minors should not be tested unless there is a medically compelling reason for doing so, i.e., an at-risk child is believed to be showing symptoms. However, under no circumstances is testing a substitute for a thorough neurological and neuropsychological workup. . . . Parental anxiety concerning a child's risk does not constitute a medically compelling reason. (HDSA 1994, 10)

In a 1995 report, the American Society of Human Genetics and the American College of Medical Genetics cited "timely medical benefit to the child" as the primary justification for genetic testing; "[s]ubstantial psychosocial benefit to the competent adolescent" might also justify testing. They concluded that "genetic testing generally should be deferred," however, if the benefits of testing "will not accrue until adulthood, as in the case of . . . adult-onset diseases." (ASHG/ACMG 1995, 1233)

Here, testing is sought by Liz, the mother of a six-year-old boy, who questions a pediatric neurologist's diagnosis of Tourette's syndrome and obsessive compulsive behavior in the child. Although the case provides no information about the basis for her skepticism, we learn that Charley's affected father was violent and abusive. Liz's life has already been profoundly affected by HD, and she may have an understandable tendency to blame Charley's disturbing, "atypical and unpredictable" behavior on that disorder.

We cannot be sure she is wrong, but the odds are against her. At first impression, the two disorders are dissimilar. Tourette's syndrome is characterized by motor and vocal tics; it may be associated with obsessive compulsive behavior and attention deficit disorder (Suchowersky 1994). Juvenile Huntington disease, in contrast, tends to be characterized by rigidity, and onset at age six would be unusual. Clarke and Bundey (1990) reported only one case of HD in which onset occurred at or before age ten in the West Midlands (U.K.) over a twenty-year period; based on data from the U.S. National Huntington Disease Roster, Hayden et al. (1985) found that onset occurred before age ten in less than 1 percent of all cases.

If Charley is tested, diagnosing him as a gene carrier exposes him to a real risk of stigmatization and rejection. One could imagine a scenario in which Liz responds negatively to the child, whom she might perceive as "just like his father," her estranged husband. (See the discussion of "preselection" in Case 15, "Jimmy.") However, if Charley is not tested, his mother may nonetheless conclude that he carries the HD mutation. On the other hand, if genetic testing reveals that he is not a gene carrier, he may experience increased affection and improved treatment from his mother.

To resolve this case, it is important to distinguish between presymptomatic testing and testing undertaken to confirm a diagnosis of HD; our majority opposes the former. The arguments for testing would be greatly strengthened if Charley were showing symptoms of HD. We know that he is at risk of early onset, given his father's age of onset and the tendency for juvenile cases with high CAG_n repeats to be inherited through the male parent. We also know that a pediatric neurologist has diagnosed his problem as Tourette's syndrome rather than HD.

A desirable intermediate step would be to obtain a second opinion.

A clinical examination should be conducted by a neurologist who is familiar with HD to determine whether Charley is showing early symptoms of that disorder. If the second neurologist confirms the first opinion, our majority concludes that the testing staff should refuse to test Charley.

On the other hand, if medical evidence suggests that Charley is suffering from juvenile-onset HD, we would not oppose genetic testing to confirm the diagnosis. That testing could eliminate the possibility of other, treatable disorders. While presymptomatic testing is not appropriate for minors, testing to confirm a diagnosis of HD after symptoms have appeared may be appropriate.

Testing may be important to ensure a correct diagnosis and appropriate treatment. Not all treatments for Tourette's syndrome are benign. Mild cases do not require medical treatment, but individuals who experience more severe symptoms may be treated with dopamine-depleting agents or neuroleptics (e.g., haloperidol) to control tics, and antidepressants to combat obsessive compulsive disorder. Side effects of these medications are a serious concern in Tourette's syndrome as in other disorders that require lifelong treatment (Suchowersky 1994). If the child is diagnosed with HD, a potentially harmful treatment for Tourette's could be discontinued, although haloperidol may also be prescribed to control HD chorea.

Case 18 Mr. and Mrs. B.

Mrs. B. is a twenty-eight-year-old married woman whose husband is at risk for HD. She has called a testing center several times to obtain information about HD and about presymptomatic testing. She has admitted that she feels her husband is showing symptoms of HD, but the couple has never made a clinic appointment for a diagnosis. One day she calls to say that she is pregnant and that they would like to come in to discuss their options.

During this visit, it becomes clear that the pregnancy was planned. Although the couple feel that the husband is showing symptoms, they decided that they wanted to try to have a baby. They agreed that they would seek prenatal testing, and they had planned to terminate the pregnancy if the fetus were found to be carrying the HD gene.

An appointment was scheduled for a neurological examination to determine whether Mr. B. was currently symptomatic; he was diagnosed with HD.

Mr. B. wished to pursue confirmatory testing. As the center's laboratory was not yet doing direct gene testing, a sample of his blood had to be sent to another laboratory for analysis and genetic confirmation of his results. The test confirmed the diagnosis of HD.

Mr. and Mrs. B. then decided that they wanted prenatal testing, and a sample was sent to the same laboratory. The laboratory sent back paperwork including a consent form that the couple was asked to sign, which stated:

> It has been explained to me and I understand that:
> This testing is to be carried out with the understanding that I plan to terminate those pregnancies in which the fetus has inherited the HD gene. This plan is being made to avoid the situation of a prenatal test being turned into a presymptomatic test.

Although the couple had discussed termination and were united in their decision to terminate, they did not feel comfortable signing this form. One reservation was that they did not, and could not, know how *they would feel if the prenatal testing indicated that their fetus carried the HD gene. The laboratory refused to analyze the sample unless this form was signed.*

Mr. and Mrs. B. insist that they have a right to choice regarding the outcome of the pregnancy and that no one has the right to impose an option on them. They fully understand the ramifications of continuing the pregnancy, and while they agree that they probably would terminate a fetus carrying the HD gene, they do not agree that they should have to sign anything, and they reserve the right to change their minds. The lab directors strongly object to doing a prenatal test that is tantamount to presymptomatic testing of a child. They want some signal that they will not be participants in a process with which they disagree.

It is important to understand the rationale for this apparently outrageous protocol at the outset. In general, asking a couple to sign the form serves to focus attention on the implications of their conduct and to call into question their commitment to termination. It may be wise to ask people to examine their decision more closely.

The ultimate rationale for this requirement, however, is rooted in a rejection of presymptomatic testing of children for a serious and untreatable disease such as HD. Our majority shares this rejection. (See Cases 13, "Mr. Crawford," and 14, "Mr. and Mrs. Anderson," as well as Corson et al. 1990.) Our working assumption is that individuals at risk should have the option of deciding for themselves as adults whether to be tested for late-onset diseases for which there is no treatment or cure, and that this decision should not be made by parents. It is significant that most adults at risk choose not to be tested (Quaid et al. 1987; Quaid and Morris 1993). However, not everyone agrees that presymptomatic HD testing of children is wrong (Sharpe 1993; Bloch and Hayden 1990; our minority). The relevance of this discussion to prenatal testing arises from the fact that prenatal testing of a fetus that is then brought to term is tantamount to presymptomatic testing of a child. The laboratory's policy of requiring a commitment to abort fetuses carrying the HD mutation is a natural extrapolation from a position shared by our majority.

On a first level, a judgment on this case is straightforward. No laboratory, or anyone else for that matter, can legally coerce someone to have an abortion. Even if the document were to have some sort of binding force—which it does not—it would be easy to ignore it as a practical matter. Asking Mr. and Mrs. B. to sign the form is simply a crude gesture insulting to them and tending to support misunderstanding of the law about abortion.

Furthermore, it is coercive. This vulnerable couple is looking for security and assurance, seeking a resolution of doubt so that they can plan for the future. The very act of signing a consent form may have effects beyond those intended. The couple may feel they have shifted the burden of proof in their decision making, making commitments they may not and need not have made. They may feel that responsibility for choice has been taken from them—a feeling they may greet with rage or joy; they may think that they are bound by the form regardless of their feelings. Thus, signing the form is itself a consequential act, whatever its precise legal force may be.

One argument that could be offered against the laboratory's policy would be to claim that it must be neutral, offering its services to anyone who requests them, and some of our consultants urge us to take that view. But we argue that testing centers may set reasonable standards of practice and may refuse to perform certain tests (see Cases 19, "Julie," and 20, "Barbara"); indeed, that is the practical outcome of our majority's rejection of the presymptomatic testing of children. In this case, however, the operative decision is being made by "the lab directors," who may well have no contact with the consultand—or indeed any clinical experience. Everyone might agree that if a laboratory had sloppy standards for practice (e.g., unreliable tests, overcharging, incorrect reporting of results) to the point of endangering consultands or consumers, that behavior should not be allowed to continue. What are the limits, if any, to a laboratory staff's adhering to what they believe is a moral stance?

One analogue for the issue confronting the laboratory can be found in the debate over prenatal testing for sex selection (See Wertz and Fletcher 1989a). Honoring requests for prenatal testing for sex selection respects the consultand's autonomy, a central goal for genetic counselors. On the other hand, sex selection utilizes genetic services for a condition that is nonmedical and for an end that many regard as reprehensible (Resta 1992). Many counselors feel extremely uncomfortable with this situation, torn between their support for a woman's right to have an abortion for any reason and their rejection of this particular reason. Usually, the decision whether to honor such a request remains in the hands of the individual counselor. Here, the issue is different, and laboratory policy has been substituted for counselor discretion.

Our resolution of this case assumes that the center and counselor agree with the laboratory that children should not be presymptomatically tested for HD. Although the testing center and the counselor may reject both the imposition of any requirement by the laboratory and this specific requirement, the disagreement is over power and means, not ends.

We believe that a laboratory may legitimately refuse to perform certain kinds of tests. For example, it might refuse to offer prenatal testing for HD on the grounds that the results of these tests might be misused. Moreover, it may have an announced policy of wanting to discourage persons from testing if they do not seriously contemplate abortion. This view is consistent with our more general views about the roles of professionals as advisers or counselors, moral agents in their own right. (See Guidelines ID, IV, and particularly VI.)

We do not think the laboratory should go beyond these broad policy positions, however. At some point it must allow discretionary judgments by counselors and centers, not to mention consultands. In our case, the laboratory might announce that its policy was to offer prenatal testing only in cases where abortion is contemplated. The counselor might spend considerable time discussing the issues of presymptomatic testing of children with Mr. and Mrs. B. But in the last analysis, this discussion may be categorized as policy and professional advice that the couple may choose to ignore. The laboratory's current ill-advised requirement should be discontinued immediately.

Case 19 Julie

Julie is a twenty-eight-year-old single woman with a college education who is at risk for HD. She initially called the testing program from her home in another part of the country. At that time, she was ineligible for participation in the testing program, which restricted testing to persons who lived within 150 miles of the testing center.

During the next year, Julie called frequently. Her demeanor on the phone was insistent and demanding, and her speech was often rambling. She reported being alienated from her family because of a family history of alcohol abuse and several instances of physical abuse. She had recently been hospitalized after striking two people in two separate incidents and was under the care of a therapist.

About a year after her first call to the testing program, Julie moved to the city in which the testing program was located. Lacking employment, she lived in a hotel for two weeks, supported by a local social service agency. Soon after her arrival, she joined the local branch of Alcoholics Anonymous (AA). In a matter of days, the clinic began to receive telephone calls from people she had met at AA who were concerned about her agitated behavior. Clinic staff recommended that callers bring her to the emergency room, but no one ever did.

Julie requested presymptomatic testing. She was scheduled to be examined in the HD clinic because clinic staff felt that she needed immediate psychiatric evaluation as well as a neurological examination. Her neurological examination was within normal limits. The psychiatrist who examined her gave her a diagnosis of histrionic personality disorder and possible bipolar disorder.

An interview using the Schedule of Affective Disorders and Schizophrenia—Lifetime Version revealed a history of bipolar disorder, alcohol abuse, anorexia and bulimia, obsessive compulsive disorder, anxiety and panic disorder, and self-injurious behavior at age twenty-four. She denied all current symptomatology.

Julie was referred for pretest counseling. She was then living in a halfway house with two recovering alcoholics with whom she did not get

*along. She had no steady job and no insurance of any kind. On each of
her first three visits, she was accompanied by a different man, each of
whom she had known for only a few days.*

This case raises an important issue, the subject of extensive discussion
within the HD testing community: whether it is ever justified to postpone or deny testing (DeGrazia 1991). Denying the test to Julie seems
paternalistic and wrong, if she has not been declared incompetent and if
the decisive point in moral analysis is preservation of the autonomy of
individual patients.

However, the professionals who are most experienced in offering
presymptomatic testing are critical of the view that patient autonomy
trumps all other considerations; their warnings are based on firsthand
knowledge of the profound effects that such testing may have on individuals and their families (Brandt et al. 1989; Meissen et al. 1988; Bloch
et al. 1992; Huggins et al. 1992; Quaid 1992). They urge caution in testing for a late-onset disorder for which there is no cure or treatment
(Chapman 1992).

Generally, it cannot be the case that professionals must offer their
services to everyone who demands them. While physicians, and by exten-
sion other professionals, might be considered morally and legally required to honor a competent patient's rational refusal of therapy, this
requirement does not extend to honoring a patient's demand for a specific therapy (Gert et al. 1994). Professionals may or may not honor patients' requests for treatment, as opposed to refusal of treatment, on the
basis of carefully considered professional judgments about the legal,
moral, and medical appropriateness of the requests.

Nor is postponing testing the same thing as refusing testing alto-
gether (which we defend in Case 20, "Barbara"). In this case, the factors
that lead to a refusal to test are subject to change with a possible improvement or disappearance of the symptoms in question. The decision
may be more accurately described as postponement of testing.

A recent survey of all centers in the United States offering presymptomatic testing for HD indicates that eighteen (69 percent) of these centers reported denying or postponing testing at least once (Quaid 1993).
Justifications for denial or postponement included inappropriate requests
for testing (e.g., to confirm a diagnosis of HD that could not be achieved
using linkage testing); other decisions to postpone were based on personal or situational factors that suggested that caution should be exercised in particular cases. In actual practice, most professionals offering
testing appear to believe that a decision to deny or postpone predictive
testing may be justified.

Some suggestions about the appropriateness of such decisions can be gleaned from the two sets of published guidelines for presymptomatic testing for HD (IHA-WFN 1990, 1994; HDSA 1989, 1994). These sets of guidelines specifically address the issue of denying or postponing testing based on information obtained during the recommended screening procedures. The HDSA guidelines cover this issue in their criteria for inclusion in testing.

The guidelines offer some generalizations about factors that may preclude individuals from fulfilling the informed consent requirement. These factors include a current diagnosis of schizophrenia, manic depression, retardation, alcoholism, or other disorder that can affect judgment. The guidelines also recommend that current risk of suicide be thoroughly evaluated for test applicants with a previous history of a suicide attempt. This evaluation should take place no later than the second visit.

Guidelines further recommend that persons who are experiencing temporary stresses be asked to delay testing until these problems have been resolved. These stresses might arise from a pregnancy, major illness, litigation such as divorce proceedings or custody determination, and other traumatic events (HDSA 1989, 6).

The HDSA guidelines for testing were revised in 1994 to incorporate changes required by the discovery of the HD gene in 1993 (HD Collaborative Research Group 1993) and in response to the HD community's conviction that the elaborate testing protocols initially developed for research needed to be evaluated as testing became more widely available. The issue of psychiatric and/or psychological screening is addressed in the revised guidelines:

> Psychological and/or psychiatric screening is still strongly recommended based on the high levels of depression found in those at risk. The risk of adverse emotional response remains the single greatest risk of the test. It is important that psychological evaluation of emotional stability not be viewed as a hurdle to be jumped in order to qualify for testing, but rather as a method of identifying persons likely to need greater emotional support in follow-up. In some instances, such as overt risk for suicide and/or major depressive symptoms, it is appropriate to delay testing, initiate psychiatric treatment, and stabilize the individual before proceeding with the test. (HDSA 1994, 9)

The International Huntington Association and World Federation of Neurology guidelines address the issue in recommendation 2.5: "For applicants with evidence of a serious previous or current psychiatric condition, it may be advisable that testing be postponed and supportive services be put in place" (IHA-WFN 1990).

On the assumption that these guidelines represent a reasonable translation of the idea that voluntary and informed consent is required before carrying out testing, let us return to the present case. The counselor has several indications that Julie might be emotionally unstable. In the course of her contact with the center over the previous year, her telephone conversations were often rambling and disconnected. Calls from people who had just met Julie at AA raised the issue of alcohol abuse, as well as behavior that disturbed strangers to the extent that they took action on their own initiative.

In addition to her possible emotional problems, the consultand's social situation is unstable. She moved to the city with no job and no money; her present living arrangements and financial situation are precarious.

Because HD first presents approximately 50 percent of the time with a psychiatric disorder, it seems possible that Julie's current symptoms indicate the onset of HD. Although her neurological findings were within normal limits, Julie's psychiatric examination, completed as part of the testing research protocol, revealed evidence of a possible bipolar disorder. In fact, her psychiatric interview revealed a lifetime history of psychological problems. It was clear that she had had a tumultuous life including a dysfunctional family, a series of abusive sexual encounters, and a record of drifting from job to job despite having a college degree. The overall impression of a highly emotional and unstable personality was reinforced by records from her former therapist, obtained with Julie's consent.

Julie has an unstable living situation and is not employed. She has no social supports and is estranged from her family of origin. She manifests psychiatric symptoms that might be the initial symptoms of HD. In these circumstances, we believe that Julie's test should be postponed. We assume that the counselor will remain in contact with Julie. If her circumstances improve, and if Julie continues to seek testing, we assume that it will be offered.

Case 20 Barbara

The consultand, Barbara, is a thirty-four-year-old single woman. At the age of two, she had an episode of encephalitis, which left her with mild neurological abnormalities and subnormal intelligence. She attended special classes all through school and obtained a high school diploma. She lives independently in subsidized housing and supports herself by caring for her mother, who has HD. Her father pays her for this work, but she has no insurance or other benefits.

The initial request for presymptomatic genetic testing in this family came from the consultand's older, married sister. The consultand accompanied this sister to her first appointment and requested testing for herself.

Barbara's neurological examination was within normal limits. Psychiatric screening revealed feelings of depression at irregular times, but she did not meet criteria for clinical depression. She was referred for pretest counseling.

Barbara had a total of four counseling sessions lasting approximately one and one-half hours each. When discussing her reasons for testing, she stated that she did not plan to change jobs, marry, or ever to have children. The counselor reviewed the inheritance of HD and the mechanics of linkage testing at every meeting, but at no point during these sessions was Barbara able to report accurately either her current risk for HD or how testing might change her knowledge of her risk. She was unable to discuss the possible social or emotional ramifications of testing. At various times during the counseling sessions, she said that perhaps it would be better not to be tested; at other times she was adamant about continuing. She kept her counseling appointments inconsistently and sometimes forgot to call to cancel a scheduled appointment.

Clinic staff were seriously concerned about Barbara's capacity to provide informed consent. A consultation was arranged with members of an ethics advisory committee formed when testing first became available. The committee concluded that Barbara did not appear to have the capac-

*ity to make an autonomous decision about testing and recommended that
testing be postponed indefinitely.*

*The clinic staff met with Barbara to discuss its reservations about
testing her and the decision to postpone testing. At the time, she did not
appear particularly disturbed by this information.*

*Three months later, after her sister received her test results, Barbara
called to say that she wanted to be tested. Three days later, the counselor
received a call from a local therapist, a social worker Barbara had started
to see as part of the testing protocol. Barbara had asked the social worker
to act as her advocate in seeking testing. The social worker volunteered
that she did not feel comfortable in that role and that she did not think
that Barbara had a clear understanding of the test or the implications of
the results. The social worker reported that she was having trouble assessing Barbara's desires with regard to testing. She agreed to try to explore
these issues in further detail.*

*Barbara has accompanied her affected parent to the HD clinic on
two occasions. She has not reiterated her request for testing.*

This case presents the issue of presymptomatic testing for a consultand
whose decision-making capacity is questionable.

According to the President's Commission for the Study of Ethical
Problems in Medicine and Biomedical and Behavioral Research, decision-making capacity requires: (1) possession of a set of values or goals;
(2) the ability to communicate and to understand information; and
(3) the ability to reason and deliberate about one's choices. Usually, three
to five criteria are offered for the assessment of these capacities: (1) ability to understand information or factual comprehension; (2) evidencing
a choice as focused on the presence or absence of a decision; (3) rational
reasoning and manipulation of information, including judgment and the
weighing of risks and benefits; (4) appreciation of the nature of the situation, including the circumstances and consequences of a decision; (5) reasonable outcome of choice (President's Commission 1982).

Barbara is described as a woman of less-than-normal intelligence
with mild neurological abnormalities, the sequelae of encephalitis in
early childhood. After approximately six hours of counseling, she cannot
describe her current risk for HD, explain how her risk status might be
clarified by testing, or discuss the emotional or social ramifications of
testing. She displays ambivalence over whether to pursue testing. Both
the counselor and the consultand are frustrated. The counselor has grave
reservations about testing Barbara, as she is convinced that Barbara does
not understand the risks and benefits of presymptomatic testing. More-

over, it seems highly possible that information will be misinterpreted if Barbara is tested. Given the difficulties of imparting information prior to testing, it may be impossible to correct these misinterpretations after testing.

One response would be simply to honor Barbara's request for testing. It is perfectly legitimate for an individual to seek testing to resolve uncertainty or simply to learn what to hope for. Although misunderstandings may occur after testing, at least the consultand will have had the test she requested. Persons with retardation are not the only persons who may misunderstand or misinterpret. Respecting a request for testing might mean a great deal in the context of a life in which autonomy has been limited.

Established guidelines for testing may recommend against proceeding in situations such as that presented by this case, however. World Federation of Neurology guidelines specify the "essential" information to be given to a consultand before presymptomatic testing for HD, including general information about HD, information about the test, information about the consequences of testing, and information on alternatives to testing. The guidelines call for an interval of three to six months with an absolute minimum of one month between the provision of this information and the actual testing; the interval is intended to allow the participant time to make an informed decision whether to proceed with testing (IHA-WFN 1990).

In general, requirements for informed consent dictate that the patient must be provided with all relevant information about the procedure and must agree voluntarily to the procedure. If the individual lacks the intellectual capacity to understand the explanations offered by medical caregivers, as in this case, she cannot provide meaningful consent.

HDSA's *Guidelines for Predictive Testing for Huntington's Disease* appear to support that conclusion. The guidelines specify:

> The criteria for inclusion in the testing program are based upon the decision that the individual for whom the test is to be performed has made an informed choice. . . . Those people considered unable to fulfill the informed choice requirement would include those with a current diagnosis of . . . retardation. (HDSA 1989, 6)

The revised guidelines state that when test results are delivered, the counselor is responsible for ascertaining "that the pretest information has been properly understood and should take the initiative to be assured of this" (HDSA 1994, 10).

A second issue concerns the voluntariness of the consultand's decision to be tested. Barbara's interest in testing may have been influenced by the fact that her older sister requested testing; she may be motivated by a desire to do something that her sister is doing. On the other hand, while other family members may have a stake in presymptomatic diagnosis of the consultand, the case offers no evidence that others are encouraging her to seek testing or requesting testing for her.

Third, Barbara has no apparent or compelling interest in testing. She has no plans for marriage or childbearing. If testing is not done, the circumstances of her life will not change significantly. If the test is done, and if the result indicates a high risk, Barbara's life may change for the worse, perhaps as a result of faulty interpretations of the results and their meaning.

We conclude that testing may be refused because of Barbara's apparently diminished capacity to provide meaningful consent, uncertainty as to her motivations and wishes, and the absence of significant reasons to pursue testing. We are troubled by this conclusion, however. This case is unique: It is the one case in which we recommend testing refusal rather than postponement. We believe that it would be appropriate for the center to arrange for Barbara to be seen by someone who is experienced in assessing the capacities of persons with mental retardation. Barbara may have been intimidated by the atmosphere of the testing center, and the counselor may not be expert in communicating with persons who have diminished capacities. The recommended consultation might or might not reverse the decision to refuse testing, but we would have more confidence in our judgment if it were done.

Case 21 Doug

Doug, a man at risk for HD, recently moved into the area, apparently to meet local test protocol requirements for the presymptomatic test. Doug, who is in his mid-thirties and is divorced, has a history of attempted suicide and penal incarceration.

The genetic counselor points out the lack of local emotional support and recommends that Doug establish a counseling relationship, either inside or outside the testing program. The counselor describes the procedures specified in the testing protocol, which include psychiatric evaluation and pre- and posttest counseling.

Doug reacts negatively and vehemently to the rigors of the test protocol and insists on being tested without undergoing the screening and evaluation procedures.

This cases raises two problems—the requirements of psychiatric evaluation and local emotional support.

Huntington disease has a profound emotional and social impact on the individual and family at risk, including depression, anxiety, and family conflict (Hayden 1981) and an increased risk of suicide (Schoenfeld et al. 1984; Farrer 1986). When presymptomatic testing for HD was initially introduced—as an experimental procedure—researchers sought ways to ensure that persons seeking testing were psychologically stable and that they would have adequate emotional and social support as they confronted the implications of their diagnoses. Testing protocols, developed with those goals in mind, are designed to evaluate the psychological and social factors that may impair adjustment to test results and to identify persons who may need assistance or treatment before testing is performed (Fox et al. 1989). Accumulating experience indicates that individuals have coped successfully with presymptomatic diagnosis in the context of testing programs that provide education, psychiatric screening, and pre- and posttest counseling (Meissen et al. 1988; Brandt et al. 1989; Huggins et al. 1992; Bloch et al. 1992).

However, critics have attacked testing protocols as rigid and paternalistic. They have characterized protocols as a series of obstacles that must be negotiated by persons who wish to learn vital information about themselves, a set of rules developed in the abstract and imposed without regard to individual circumstances. A specific objection relates to the cost of pretest screening and counseling, which may preclude testing for persons with limited means.

This debate is occurring in a setting of heightened emphasis on patient autonomy (Faden and Beauchamp 1986; Katz 1984). Successful malpractice litigation has penalized health care providers who have failed to provide adequate information that would enable patients to make fully informed decisions. Tracing the history of litigation in this area, Pelias (1991) describes an expanded conception of physicians' responsibility, which includes the duty to inform patients about their diagnoses, proposed treatments and the risks associated with them, and alternative therapies. Disclosure is intended to enhance patients' ability to make fully informed decisions about their own care. Citing professional norms of nondirective counseling, Pelias argues that genetic counselors may risk legal liability and damage the credibility of their profession if they fail to provide complete information to patients.

In Case 19, "Julie," testing was postponed because of the consult-and's lack of family and social supports, lifetime history of psychological problems, erratic behavior, unstable living situation, suggestions of alcohol abuse, and possible psychiatric symptoms. As noted in the discussion of that case, one reason for the decision to postpone testing was to provide the counseling team with an opportunity for further evaluation of the consultand's psychiatric condition. Here, in contrast, the consultand is challenging the legitimacy of the evaluation process itself.

Psychiatric assessment seems entirely warranted in this case. As noted, an elevated risk of suicide has been defined for persons diagnosed with HD; the risk appears particularly acute for Doug, who has an actual history of attempted suicide. The testing program clearly has a moral responsibility to assess Doug's current state of emotional health before proceeding (Smurl and Weaver 1987; HDSA 1989; IHA-WFN 1990).

HDSA's revised guidelines address this point explicitly.

> The risk of adverse emotional response remains the single greatest risk of the test. It is important that psychological evaluation of emotional stability not be viewed as a hurdle to be jumped in order to qualify for testing, but rather as a method of identifying persons likely to need greater emotional support in follow-up. In some instances, such as overt risk for suicide and/or major depressive symptoms, it is appropriate to delay testing, initiate psychiatric treat-

ment, and stabilize the individual before proceeding with the test.
(1994, 9)

An opposing point of view attacks this approach as paternalistic,
arguing that the appropriate course of action is to inform the consultand
of the full range of emotional and psychological risks and obtain informed consent. The argument assumes that Doug's decision-making capacity is unimpaired and asserts, "Testing delayed is testing denied."

However, presymptomatic testing in this case does not conform to
traditional physician-patient models in which the physician lays out the
risks and benefits of alternative therapies and the informed patient, col-
laborating to varying degrees with the physician, determines what course
will be pursued (Emanuel and Emanuel 1992). Here, the risks to the individual patient are unknown; psychiatric assessment is an indispensable
tool for carefully defining those risks. Analogously, a physician would
not schedule surgery without thorough testing to rule out cardiovascular
problems that could jeopardize a patient's well-being.

It is essential to note that the issue presented by this case is not
refusal of testing or even the suggestion that testing be postponed for
any significant period. This consultand refuses examinations that are
necessary in order to determine whether testing is appropriate. Were
Doug to be examined, he might be found to be at risk for suicide or depression; postponement might then be appropriate (IHA-WFN 1990;
HDSA 1989; DeGrazia 1991), and he could be referred for preliminary
psychiatric or other treatment. On the other hand, the examination may
suggest that it is appropriate to proceed directly to testing. In that case,
the process could begin immediately. As in Case 19, "Julie," testing is
not permanently precluded, and the facts of the case reveal no circumstances that create an urgent need for immediate testing.

We conclude that counselors must not be forced to offer testing
without an adequate preliminary evaluation, but we are less supportive
of this clinic's requirement bearing on "adequate local emotional support." The consultand is divorced and has moved to the area only recently; the implication is that the individual has not had time to establish
supportive relationships.

Existing guidelines stress the desirability for candidates for testing
to select a partner to accompany them through the testing process; the
partner may be a spouse, friend, therapist, or social worker (IHA-WFN
1990; HDSA 1989). An additional suggestion is that the candidate identify local counseling support in addition to that offered by the testing
center (HDSA 1989).

Important as personal support may be, in the current case, the presence or absence of a partner alone should not be dispositive. At a minimum, Doug could establish a supportive relationship with the counselor attached to the testing program, who should be prepared to offer support throughout the testing process and its aftermath (IHA-WFN 1990). In addition, Doug might be referred to a local lay support group or a counselor or therapist. The fact that he is unwilling to identify a companion is not a sufficient reason for refusing the test.

Case 22 *Uncle Lee*

Lee S. presented at forty-seven years of age with end-stage renal disease secondary to autosomal dominant polycystic kidney disease, diagnosed by intravenous pyelogram at age forty. Renal transplantation is the treatment of choice for ESRD in ADPKD. Relatives are preferred as organ donors due to their availability and the somewhat improved transplant outcome rate. Lee's only unaffected child (age eight) was too young to volunteer as a donor. Therefore, Lee approached the children of his brother, Bill, who also had ADPKD (see pedigree) to ask that they participate in linkage studies to determine their gene status and suitability as potential organ donors.

Two of Bill's children (Jeff and Kevin), ages twenty-four and twenty-one, respectively, were eligible to be kidney donors. Neither showed symptoms, and Kevin had had a normal renal ultrasound two years previously. A third sibling had ADPKD; Bill's fourth child, Susan, had already donated a kidney to her father. DNA analysis was recommended by the Genetics Division because of the risk of false negative ultrasound results in at-risk individuals in this age range.

Blood samples were obtained from eleven family members. Linkage analysis indicated a 94 percent probability that Jeff had inherited the ADPKD gene, while Susan and Kevin appeared not to have inherited this gene. Ultrasonography later confirmed that Jeff had ADPKD. Kevin was relieved that he was unaffected, but he was ambivalent about organ donation to his Uncle Lee, and he did not volunteer his test results to his family. Lee and his wife contacted the genetics program directly to request the test results so that they could discuss the possibility of organ donation with their nephews.

After undergoing linkage testing, Kevin is relieved to learn that he will not develop ADPKD, but he now confronts pressure to donate a kidney to his uncle. He may prefer to donate a kidney to one of his two siblings or decline to serve as a donor. Kevin feels ambivalent and pressured by various family members, and he wants to keep his genetic status private.

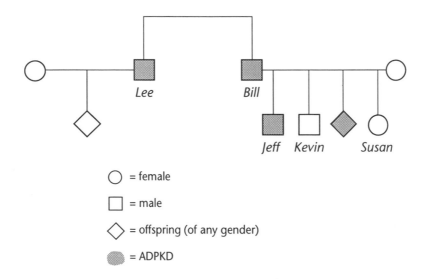

○ = female

☐ = male

◇ = offspring (of any gender)

● = ADPKD

Informed consent requires understanding and voluntariness. In this case, Kevin might consent to two separate procedures: genetic testing and organ donation. Neither is a therapeutic procedure for him. The first consent is for gene testing. The consultand must understand the risks, benefits, and alternatives for both presymptomatic testing and organ donation; the possibility of family manipulation must be discussed with the consultand (Faden and Beauchamp 1986). Because that possibility is one of the risks for Kevin in participating in the testing program, he cannot be said to have given an informed consent if he was not made aware of the possibility.

Consent for genetic testing must be clearly separated from consent for organ donation. Kevin could consent to undergo genetic testing and subsequently decide not to donate. Thus, the genetic testing program should obtain consent only for genetic testing; after appropriate pre- and posttest counseling, the consultand will have an opportunity to discuss consent for organ donation with a surgeon and others if applicable.

In actual practice Kevin may find it much harder to separate the two issues than this analysis suggests. For example, if his brother Jeff has informed Uncle Lee of his result, Kevin will find it virtually impossible not to disclose his status. If he discloses, he will encounter significant pressure to donate a kidney. To be sure, good clinical advice may minimize this problem: Kevin is not an optimal match for Uncle Lee, and results from unrelated cadaver donors may be almost as good. But many people die awaiting a transplant, and Uncle Lee and his wife are obviously desperate. Kevin's possible preference for reserving his kidney for

Jeff (for whom he will probably provide a better match), or not to donate at all, are likely to be portrayed in the family as selfish or cowardly in the face of Uncle Lee's immediate danger. Kevin is faced with an uncle who needs a kidney now and two siblings who will require a kidney in the future. How can he reconcile these competing claims and duties?

Fortunately, the genetic counselor does not have to resolve that problem, but she must help him see it, and she can help him out in certain ways. First she should honor his request that his genetic status not be revealed to anyone. Indeed, that should have been the publicly stated terms of the testing protocol from the program's inception. A genetics testing program related to the possibility of organ transplantation should anticipate this kind of outcome and should have procedures in place to ensure each individual's confidentiality. Ideally, pretest counseling would advise both Jeff and Kevin to keep to themselves the fact that they are undergoing presymptomatic testing, let alone the results of the test—unless one of them should choose to donate. There can be no question of the counselor honoring Uncle Lee's request for information about his nephew. Jeff and Kevin should be able to be tested for ADPKD without the knowledge of other family members and without disclosing their genetic status (Frankel and Teich 1993).

Suppose, however, that the family is aware of Jeff's test results, and Kevin does not want to donate a kidney. Should the counselor help to shield him from family pressure, perhaps by saying for the record that he is not a *suitable* donor—leaving the exact reasons for his unsuitability vague? That would not be a lie, as psychological factors are legitimately related to the issue of donor suitability. We reluctantly accept this option, but we are troubled by the dissembling involved, and we think it is highly preferable for confidentiality to be strictly maintained so that the counselor can hold to a policy of strict candor.

Case 23 Emily

Emily, the consultand, is a thirty-two-year-old married woman referred for presymptomatic testing because of a family history of Huntington disease.

When Emily called the testing center for her first appointment, she refused to give the secretary her address and telephone number. Instead she called back several times until she reached the counselor directly. She asked to see the counselor in her private office instead of the clinic space where patients are normally seen because she knows people who work at the hospital and wished to avoid the lobby and other public areas. At the beginning of the first interview, Emily explained that she wanted absolute confidentiality regarding her case. She was assured that that was the usual policy, and that the center would comply carefully with her request.

Emily stated that she was in good health. She had no obvious signs of HD. She wanted to know whether she had the gene for HD before becoming pregnant. She felt the situation was urgent because her unaffected paternal grandfather was very old and in precarious health. Her affected father and his affected sibling were also in poor health. She wanted blood samples taken from these individuals as soon as possible.

Emily stated that her affected father lives alone at home where he is cared for by a home health aide paid for by "the family." Her mother is living. However, Emily's parents were divorced after her father developed symptoms of HD but before he was diagnosed. There had been several incorrect diagnoses over a period of several years before her father was told he had HD by a neurologist who was treating the father's brother. As the oldest daughter of divorced parents, Emily apparently played a primary role in her father's quest for a diagnosis, and she is the only member of her immediate family who knows her father's diagnosis.

Emily and her husband have been married for six years. She describes her life as "perfect" and does not want to disrupt it by informing her husband that she is at 50 percent risk for HD. She has two younger unmarried sisters who, because they do not know their father's diagnosis, do not know their own risk. She sees no reason for their lives to be *disturbed now, but plans to tell them "when necessary." She does not want to inform her mother until one of her sisters "gets it." She sees no reason to worry her in the interim. She has not told her husband because she can foresee that he will be very upset. When asked to predict her husband's reaction at some time in the future, when he learns about the family history and her prior knowledge, she replies, "He'll be angry." She refused to consider the implications of deciding not to become pregnant if the presymptomatic test is positive. Presumably she would not tell her husband why she did not want to have children. She stated, "I can handle that."*

Trust and credibility mattered less to Emily than the impact on the lives of her close family members of learning about the risk for HD. She predicted that informing her family of her risk would be "like I had HD from that time on and would ruin all the years between informing and becoming symptomatic." She volunteered that she will not kill herself if she finds out she is at risk. She explained, "When I got my father's diagnosis, that was it. This is nothing. It's all or nothing. Either you're at risk or you're not." If she develops HD, she plans to divorce her husband, live alone with a paid companion, and allow her husband to visit her if he wishes to do so.

The counselor explained the patient protocol for presymptomatic testing. The constraints Emily wished to impose created several problems. She was unwilling either to designate a companion for the required visits or to obtain blood samples from her mother and sisters for linkage studies once she was told they would have to be informed of the nature of the test.

The counselor struck a bargain with Emily. She agreed to take blood samples from affected family members and the patient's paternal grandfather. The idea was to analyze the samples to see whether the family was informative with samples from just those people. If the family is uninformative on the basis of these samples, Emily would have to make a decision about including her mother and sisters. If it is informative, she will have to decide how to comply with the terms of the protocol with regard to a companion for the protocol period. Further counseling was planned after these initial test results. Emily is privately paying for these tests and the counseling visit.

Emily asked that messages be left for her at a designated telephone number. She said she would get the messages by the following day and call the counselor. It became apparent that the person with whom messages were left was her father's home health aide; her father's explosive speech was audible in the background. Emily never revealed her married name, address, or telephone number.

As it turns out, the samples submitted by Emily's family members enabled the clinic to conduct linkage testing for Emily. Emily once returned a call to arrange for a visit to obtain and discuss the results, but this attempt at contact failed, and she has not called back again.

Emily's extreme concern for confidentiality coupled with her willingness to deceive her family called her credibility into question with the counselor. Should the counselor have struck this bargain with her? If she agrees to bring a companion, should she be trusted to comply with all the visits required following testing? Should the clinic refuse a presymptomatic test in this situation?

This case, dating from the era of linkage testing for HD, revolves around the consultand's request to be tested "off protocol." In this case, a secretive consultand asked to meet the counselor in a private office instead of the usual clinic location because of concern about confidentiality. In addition, the consultand did not want to bring a confidant with her for support, although the testing protocol recommends a testing partner (IHA-WFN 1990, HDSA 1989). Finally, Emily refused to discuss important implications of testing, especially the importance of informing family members about their risk of HD and her request for presymptomatic testing.

Emily immediately aroused the counselor's suspicion when she requested a private meeting instead of the usual office appointment. In an attempt to reassure her about confidentiality, the counselor agreed to this request. Emily understands confidentiality to mean that *no one* else will know that she is at risk or that she is seeking presymptomatic testing. What is most troubling is that her secrecy extends to her husband, her mother, and her sisters.

The counselor understands confidentiality as part of her professional obligation, primarily to protect the consultand; assured confidentiality also encourages persons to seek testing and serves to protect other family members. But a professional commitment to confidentiality does not mean that the counselor always thinks that the consultand should keep the testing process secret. Like the consultand in Case 7, "Robert," Emily doesn't want to inform obviously concerned family members despite the fact that she is seeking a genetic test with profound implications for them (Hayes 1992). The issue is not the possibility that the counselor will inform those persons, but her conviction that the consultand may have a moral responsibility to do so. The great dissonance between the perspectives of counselor and consultand on this issue portends a lengthy and arduous pretest counseling relationship.

Once again, this case emphasizes the importance of the counseling process. Skillful counseling ensures informed consent before the test and then helps consultands deal with their test results. Pretest counseling fits the model of informed consent for a complicated medical procedure in which the counselor clarifies the risks, benefits and alternatives to testing. On the other hand, posttest counseling often demands skillful therapy to help the consultand and others cope with the test results.

The consultand should understand the implications of presymptomatic testing for other family members. The counselor's primary duty is to the consultand, but it does not stop there. The duty to other family members requires the counselor to inform the consultand about how her decision to be tested might affect each of them. In Emily's case, the counselor is obligated to satisfy the requirements of informed consent as fully as possible before the test and then to be available for or arrange for effective posttest counseling. It may take the counselor a great deal of time to become convinced that the consultand understands the risks and benefits of presymptomatic testing. Testing, whether it confirms the presence or absence of the HD gene, may have powerful effects on both the consultand and others (Wiggins et al. 1992; Chapman 1992; Bloch et al. 1992; Huggins et al. 1992).

Although present guidelines clearly specify the need for a counseling partner, having such a partner is best seen as a means to an end, as we argue in Case 21, "Doug." A testing partner or confidant is probably less important than a commitment by the consultand and the counselor to meet regularly for follow-up after the test results are known. This protocol requirement should be treated as a guideline, not as an inflexible rule.

In our view the counselor was right to strike the bargain that she did with Emily. She needs to explore Emily's reasons for seeking testing in greater depth—but once these reasons have been fully explored and understood, the counselor should not refuse testing based solely on the consultand's reasons for wanting to be tested. Nor should the counselor refuse to test Emily because she declines to bring a testing partner.

Once counseling has begun, the counselor is obliged to probe Emily's reasons for testing in order to make certain that she is adequately informed. Emily's reasons for testing are highly relevant to the content of these counseling sessions, less relevant on the issue of access to testing. The counselor must discuss at length Emily's responsibility to inform other concerned family members. Ultimately, Emily's request for testing should be honored, even if she continues to insist on the exclusion of her husband, mother, and sisters from knowledge of this endeavor.

Case 24 Mrs. K.

Mrs. K, a forty-two-year-old woman at risk for Huntington disease, is married and has two children, ages twenty-three and eighteen. Her father, two paternal uncles, and one paternal aunt are living and affected with HD. Her paternal grandmother, one paternal aunt, and one paternal uncle died of the disease. Her mother and paternal grandfather are alive and healthy.

Mrs. K. came to the area from out of state for testing. She was very well informed about HD; she had gathered blood from family members years ago for research purposes. She and her husband were determined to learn whether she had the gene. During counseling, they raised questions about the inflexibility of the program. They said that they had spent the last twenty-three years thinking about the issues involved in testing, and they were sure of their decision. They both stated that they felt strongly that they should not have to have expensive testing and counseling sessions from which they had nothing to gain. They felt that they had to convince the clinic staff of their decision.

More straightforward than Case 23, "Emily," this case also challenges a testing protocol. The consultand requests that certain protocol requirements be waived. Usually, the first counseling appointment requires one to two hours of genetic counseling and one hour of psychosocial evaluation (HDSA 1989). This consultand may require less than one hour of genetic counseling but perhaps the full hour of psychosocial evaluation. If the consultand is as well informed about HD as she appears to be, and if she satisfies the counselor's concerns, the required second and third visits could be collapsed into her first visit. This session would include a neurological examination, review of medical records, review of family DNA analysis, and obtaining a blood sample from the consultand.

The consultand could then return in ten to fourteen days to receive her test result and additional counseling, which normally is not done until the fourth visit. Her second visit may require one to two hours. If the consultand has a positive result, the counselor will call her by telephone the next day to reaffirm support and assistance, offer counseling if needed, and set a date for a follow-up visit. The consultand will be scheduled to return to the testing center at two months, six months, one year, eighteen months, and two years after testing (HDSA 1989). These follow-up visits cannot be forced, but they are strongly encouraged. In this case, follow-up with the patient's local physician and counselor might suffice.

This case emphasizes the importance of the counseling process and the difference between pre- and posttest counseling. The goals of counseling before testing include giving the patient enough information to make an informed decision about whether she wants to be tested. After testing, however, the counseling process becomes more like therapy. The counselor must help the consultand cope with the test results and adapt to certain knowledge of her gene status. Pretest counseling requires sharing information with the consultand to obtain informed consent; posttest counseling, in contrast, requires the counselor to help the consultand deal with the outcome of testing. Pretest counseling only begins the process that posttest counseling helps complete.

We conclude that a testing center, in rare circumstances such as this case, could collapse several appointments to assist a well-informed consultand's effort to save time and money. The center should not eliminate counseling, but it should be prepared to shorten the process significantly if circumstances warrant. In some cases the consultand will not need four appointments to accomplish the objectives of the testing program. The program requires that the consultand be at risk for HD, well-informed before testing, asymptomatic, and properly counseled. Informed consent to testing requires that the consultand understand the risks, benefits, and alternatives to testing and that she voluntarily agree to be tested. These objectives and requirements can sometimes be satisfied without rigid adherence to the letter of the testing protocol.

Case 25 Ruth

*Ruth, a forty-one-year-old woman whose deceased mother was diag-
nosed with Huntington disease, sought predictive testing. Her father and
three at-risk siblings were available for testing. Ruth had no children. In
the preceding year, she had had two pregnancies, both of which resulted
in a fetus with trisomy 21 and were terminated. During the last pregnancy, Ruth and her husband opted for prenatal exclusion testing, and
studies were initiated on the consultand, her father, and her three siblings.
Studies were not done on the fetus because of the diagnosis of Down syndrome.*

*Results of the haplotype testing were made available to the clinic
staff prior to initiating the predictive testing protocol. Ruth was not
aware of the results. The studies revealed that one sibling had the same
haplotype as Ruth; the other two siblings shared an identical haplotype,
which differed from Ruth's.*

*Early in the protocol Ruth indicated that two of her siblings had ex-
hibited obvious signs of HD for several years. The clinic staff had reason
to regard this information as accurate, and they knew that these siblings
were the two whose haplotype differed from Ruth's. One brother was reportedly told by his internist that he appeared to have HD. However, the
brother would not release this information and, therefore, it could not be
confirmed. He also indicated he would not pursue formal neurological
evaluation.*

*If the clinical information provided by Ruth was correct, the staff
knew the HD status of all the siblings in this family including the consult-
and (i.e., if one of the two siblings with a haplotype that differed from
Ruth's haplotype had HD, then Ruth did not carry the gene).*

*Ruth strongly desired a pregnancy. She wanted prenatal exclusion
testing if she became pregnant again and if predictive testing were not
possible.*

This case raises the question of what counselors ought to do when
they have haplotype information plus credible, but unconfirmed, clini-

cal information that suggests that a consultand does not carry the HD gene.

As this case is written, it is unclear whether any of the results of haplotype testing may be shared with Ruth, for example, that her haplotype differs from those of one or more of her named siblings. The extent to which that information is confidential should be specified in the informed consent to the original test. It is certainly arguable that no information about the haplotypes of any members of her family should ever be shared with Ruth. But it is understandable that this prohibition has not and will not always be observed, especially in the course of linkage studies. We proceed on the assumption that the terms of the original consent allow the counselor to inform Ruth that her haplotype differs from that of X, Y, or Z sibling, and that Ruth has already been so informed.

With no information except her mother's diagnosis, Ruth's risk would have been 50 percent, and her potential offspring's risk would have been 25 percent. If her report about her siblings is correct, the haplotype information reduces those risks substantially, although it cannot completely eliminate them. Somehow, perhaps through personal observation of the siblings, the clinic has "reason to regard this information as accurate." It is not sensible to behave as if the unconfirmed observations are worthless.

If neither sibling agrees to neurological testing to confirm the diagnosis of HD, we believe the counselors should tell Ruth that, *if* her reports about her siblings are correct, the chance of her carrying the HD gene is very small. The counselor should accurately report the results of the testing that has been undertaken and discuss the inferences that *may* follow from those results. By telling Ruth what they know, the counselors can increase her information and offer her significant reassurance. They must not pretend to a greater level of certainty than they can have. They must emphasis that their knowledge takes the conditional form of "If X, then not Y."

What if the counselors were less confident of the unconfirmed information? Simply assuming the truth of hearsay information could be very dangerous, because Ruth contemplates serious—indeed, life-changing—actions. Again, the answer seems relatively straightforward: The counselors should summarize the information that is known, including the uncertainties. We do not recommend freewheeling speculation. If the counselors do not think the hearsay information deserves any weight, then they have no information to convey. If counselors have no information, they should not tell Ruth something that is both meaningless and confusing. Discretion in making these judgment calls should be part of the skills of a good counselor.

Case 26 Jackie

The coordinator of a testing center receives a call from a young man inquiring about testing. He says he is calling on behalf of Jackie, a young woman at risk for HD, who wants to know whether she carries the gene for HD. However, Jackie works for an insurance company and is very concerned about the effect on her career if information about her test result were ever revealed. Therefore, she would like to go through testing anonymously: She is willing to come in person to the testing center for a neurological examination and for pretest counseling, but she is not willing to reveal her identity.

The counselor is aware of the potential negative impact of third parties' access to genetic information, and she understands Jackie's concerns. She is also aware that the issue of anonymous testing is one that has been raised within the genetics community and is one that must be addressed. After discussing the issue, the counselor and the neurologist agree that they will try to work with Jackie to determine whether anonymous testing is feasible.

Jackie comes to the testing center with her male friend, Tom. She refuses to reveal her last name, phone number, or address. Her neurological examination is normal, and she is referred for pretest counseling.

During the first counseling session, the counselor asks some standard questions regarding the family history of the disorder and whether any samples are available from an affected relative. Jackie's knowledge of her family history is sketchy. Without a last name, the counselor is unable to check the testing center's database of HD families for evidence of family history or banked tissue samples. The counselor feels that she must confirm a family history of HD and asks Jackie to arrange for her affected mother's medical records to be sent to the center.

Jackie believes that her mother's medical records will reveal her last name and thus her identity. She insists on trying to have the medical records sent directly to her so that she can erase any identifying information before sending the records on to the center. Not surprisingly, the health

*care center refuses to send the medical records directly to Jackie. It ap-
pears that no medical records will be forthcoming.*

*Jackie continues to refuse to reveal her phone number or address.
To communicate with her, the counselor must call Tom at work and leave
a message. Tom then calls Jackie, and Jackie calls the counselor at home
in the evening. This indirect communication is increasingly frustrating,
and the counselor feels that it is a great hindrance to proper handling of
the case.*

*The counselor feels uncomfortable. She must establish a family his-
tory of HD to enable a correct interpretation of Jackie's test. Without
a sample of tissue from an affected relative, there is no way to rule out
other disorders. Without medical records, there is no way of determining
the medical history and course of the disease in the family. The counselor
is uncertain how to proceed. She tells Jackie that she wishes to talk to her
colleagues in order to decide what to do next.*

*Three days later the counselor returns home late in the evening. Her
husband says that someone has been calling every five or ten minutes and
hanging up on the answering machine. When he answered the phone, a
woman asked for the counselor. He says that the woman sounded upset
and was crying. He told the woman that he expected the counselor home
any minute. The woman said that she would call back in ten or fifteen
minutes, but she would not leave her number.*

*The counselor is concerned and wonders which of her consultands
might be calling. She waits up for a return call, but no one ever calls.*

*The next day, Tom calls to say that Jackie is upset because she does
not know whether the counselor is ever going to test her. He will not confirm that Jackie called the counselor the night before, but he does not
deny it. The counselor explains that she wants to try to work with Jackie
but that she feels she must do several things in order to do her job properly and that Jackie's desire to remain anonymous is making these things
impossible. Tom becomes quite insistent. He says that his job is to solve
problems, and he wants to do whatever it takes to get Jackie tested. Tom
wants to know exactly what the counselor needs before she will agree to
test Jackie.*

What should the counselor do?

In Case 12, "Mr. L.," we noted that persons who seek testing for genetic
diseases have legitimate concerns about their insurability. Billings et al.
(1992), Barash (1994), and Geller et al. (1996) have described instances
of genetic discrimination reported by applicants for health, life, and disability insurance. We can understand why the counselor in this case
agrees with the consultand that the issue is serious and real.

In Case 23, "Emily," the consultand sought anonymous testing in order to "protect" other family members from the facts that her father had been diagnosed with Huntington disease, and that she and her sisters were at risk. Here, in contrast, the consultand wants to avoid disclosing information about herself to her employer, an insurance company.

In the present case, the counselor has agreed to explore the feasibility of anonymous testing. Anonymous testing has been widely used for HIV, and at least one center has experimented with it for HD, but it presents at least two problems. First, in situations in which helpful medical interventions are possible, anonymity makes it difficult if not impossible for a health care provider to offer treatment.

Second, mistakes about the nature of a genetic disease are common. Families that think they have HD may, in fact, have a different problem. Families may believe that they are at risk of HD, when they are actually at risk of other neurological disorders, some involving CAG repeats (e.g., dentatorubral pallidolusyian atrophy). If Jackie is tested anonymously, there is a chance of concluding that she is not at risk for HD, but there is no way to rule out her risk for another neurological disorder that runs in her family. Thus, Jackie's desire for anonymity presents a practical problem for HD testing: The counselor has no way of confirming that she is actually at risk for HD. Although Jackie reports that her mother is affected, the counselor can't obtain medical records that support the diagnosis. Without the mother's name, which Jackie refuses to provide, the counselor cannot determine whether information or a tissue sample is available through the HD data bank. From the counselor's point of view, it would be irresponsible to proceed with testing without a confirmed diagnosis. Jackie and the counselor have reached a stalemate.

With the advent of direct testing, it may seem that information about or samples from other family members are not needed. If Jackie were tested, and if her results revealed 40 or more CAG repeats, it would be clear that she carries the gene for HD. However, two other outcomes are possible, and a confirmed diagnosis of HD in the family history would be helpful in both cases.

First, Jackie's test might produce CAG repeats in the intermediate range (36 to 39). In that case, a confirmed diagnosis of HD in Jackie's mother, along with the number of her mother's CAG repeats, could provide additional information about Jackie's risk of developing HD. If Jackie's mother is indeed affected, and if she has a CAG repeat that is equal to Jackie's intermediate CAG repeat, that fact would increase the likelihood that Jackie will develop HD.

The second possibility is that Jackie's test will reveal a low CAG number (less than 26), which would indicate that she will not develop

HD. However, without a confirmed diagnosis of HD in Jackie's mother, the counselor cannot rule out the possibility that her mother's symptoms are caused by another neurological disorder, and she cannot assure Jackie that she will not develop symptoms of that disorder at some later date.

The initial agreement was to "try" to conduct anonymous testing. As pretest counseling has proceeded, however, it has become evident that the only kind of test that can be performed anonymously is one that is seriously flawed. It may be possible to give Jackie a definitive diagnosis of HD; it will certainly not be possible to tell her that she is not at risk for another familial neurodegenerative disorder.

As a professional, the counselor is not obligated to conduct testing under any terms that may be imposed by consultands. Rather, she is ethically obligated to exercise professional judgment and to perform competently in responding to consultands' requests. In this case, given the difficulties associated with accurate interpretation of Jackie's test results, she should not proceed with testing now.

However, the counselor should continue to work with Jackie to attempt to resolve the issues so that she can be tested. A major problem is Jackie's fear that confidentiality will not be maintained. The counselor can describe the procedures that safeguard confidential information about HD families, and she can reassure Jackie that third parties, including her employer, cannot gain access to information about her test results without her permission. The counselor must make every effort to establish a relationship of trust with the consultand and to restore her confidence in the testing center's determination and ability to protect her privacy.

A secondary problem raised by this case is Jackie's insistence on circuitous communication. Phoning the counselor at home at five- or ten-minute intervals is an abuse of the counseling relationship and an imposition on the counselor. The counselor can support and assist Jackie while maintaining appropriate professional distance and without opening herself to unreasonable demands.

Case 27 Aunt Mary

Mrs. G. is a forty-year-old woman at risk for HD. She requests linkage testing primarily for the benefit of her two children, who are entering their late teens and have expressed some concern about their risk. Blood samples are obtained from Mrs. G's affected mother and father and from one affected and two unaffected aunts and uncles. One unaffected aunt— Aunt Mary—refuses to give a blood sample. Linkage testing is done using the available samples, but it is uninformative. A blood sample is needed from Aunt Mary, but she again refuses. Both Mrs. G. and her daughter call and write Aunt Mary, to no avail.

Several months later, Mrs. G. calls the testing center to say that her aunt has been hospitalized and is not expected to live. Mrs. G asks the center staff to explain the need for a blood sample to the hospital personnel. The testing center calls the physician in charge, who readily agrees to draw blood. The center discusses with him Aunt Mary's previous refusal and the need for informed consent. A blood kit, including a consent form, is sent to the hospital. Several days later three tubes of blood, but no consent form, arrive at the center. Two days later Aunt Mary dies.

Should Aunt Mary's sample be used?

Absence of a consent form does not settle this case. A first step is to determine whether the aunt, on her deathbed, validly consented to have blood sent to the HD testing center but—for some reason—was unable to sign the consent form. Or perhaps the consent form was misplaced and simply not copied for return to the HD program. Even though these possibilities are unlikely, the testing center should contact the physician to determine whether the patient consented to the test, either orally or in writing. There is no need to be excessively scrupulous in these procedures. If a valid written consent was obtained and documented, or if the physician states that the patient gave oral consent but was unable to sign the consent form, the sample may be used. However, if the staff believes that Aunt Mary did not agree to testing or that the physician did not obtain a valid consent, or if the physician states that the patient was not asked to consent or was unable to consent, the samples must not be used.

On the basis of a brief history, we cannot know why Aunt Mary refused to cooperate, but she did—on several occasions and after several requests. Her choices may have been inspired by fear, ignorance, or revenge for real or imagined wrongs. Her reasons may have been reasonable or spiteful. In any case, her choices should have great weight. The availability of a direct gene test for HD makes the case less important for HD (but see the discussion of the ongoing importance of family in Case 26, "Jackie"), but its relevance to linkage testing in the context of other genetic disorders is obvious.

Two slight changes in this case might affect our conclusion. First, if Aunt Mary had never been asked for a sample—that is, if she had not repeatedly and clearly refused to provide one—it seems plausible to us to presume her consent and, after she is no longer competent, to use adventitiously collected blood to run the test. If we really were in doubt about Aunt Mary's wishes, there would be no reason to assume her unwillingness.

The second possibility is that a sample is drawn after Aunt Mary's death. Can the next-of-kin consent to use of her tissues after she is dead? Legally, her next-of-kin can consent to autopsy and make funeral arrangements; they may decide about organ donation unless she left explicit directions on this issue before her death.

The analogy with organ donation is instructive but imperfect. Aunt Mary did leave explicit instructions. Moreover, familial consent to organ donation is usually altruistic: The family agrees to donate organs for the benefit of others. Familial consent to use of Aunt Mary's sample, in contrast, would be self-interested. Thus, in this case, even more than in organ donation, the family's authority should not extend to the use of Aunt Mary's blood obtained after her death, especially if it is used for a purpose that she explicitly refused during her life.

Sad as this family history of alienation is, the overriding consideration is Aunt Mary's wishes, not the time at which the sample was collected. If Aunt Mary were asked on her deathbed and remained adamant, her refusal must be respected postmortem; if she were asked whether she objected to use of her sample after her death, she might have changed her mind. If so, of course, a postmortem sample may be used.

But those are not the facts in this case. Even if an argument sometimes can be made for overriding an individual's refusal to cooperate, we must be able to assure persons who seek testing of the central requirements of consent and confidentiality. Absent credible grounds for believing that Aunt Mary changed her mind, her sample should not be used.

Case 28 Scott

Scott, a man at risk for HD, calls a counselor at a large research center and expresses an interest in nondisclosing prenatal testing. When she hears his name, the counselor recognizes the surname of a large family that had participated in the early linkage studies of HD. To determine whether blood samples are available, the counselor looks up a copy of the family's pedigree, which contains preliminary linkage results. These results indicate that Scott is not the biological child of his affected father. The counselor wonders how to proceed. To inform Scott about his nonpaternity seems wrong, especially since that information was gathered during a research project. To pretend that the information does not exist and subject Scott and his wife to the physical and emotional risks of prenatal testing also seems wrong.

This case presented the counselor with two ethical dilemmas. First, she had to decide whether to look up the original pedigree and linkage results. Second, once she had looked them up, she had to decide what to do with the information they reveal. That problem, in turn, raises two different issues: (1) what to do with arguably improperly obtained information, and (2) what to do about information that reveals nonpaternity.

The case does not reveal what the family was told about confidentiality and possible uses of their blood samples when they participated in the early linkage studies, or how the informed consent forms they signed handled the issue. We assume that they were told that the studies were for research, not clinical purposes, and that all information would remain confidential, and that they agreed to those provisions. If that is correct, then the counselor should not have looked up the pedigree and linkage information for a clearly clinical purpose.

It is tempting to justify the counselor's behavior in seeking the information because she had good motives for doing so. Indeed, one member of our group thinks that the counselor's original behavior was proper. The majority, however, think that the counselor should not have checked the records. The pedigree records existed only because of the relatives' willingness to participate in a research study. For all we know, some or all of the family members may have been unwilling to participate in the original study if they had thought that any of the information or samples they provided might be used in a clinical setting.

This case might be discussed in terms of promise breaking. The reason that issues of promise breaking arise in any context is that keeping a promise is often difficult, inefficient, and wasteful. Nonetheless, there are good reasons to keep promises. One reason is fidelity, a notion rooted in respect for human beings. Another is utility: If people fail to keep promises, it will be impossible to maintain social interaction, which depends on trust. People will refuse to participate in research, for example. Like all general duties, the obligation to keep promises cannot be absolute. Here, however, the pressures to break a promise are no greater than the kind of pressures one normally envisions in deciding that promises should usually be kept.

Of course, it is possible that a counselor will remember the family's results from the research study without looking them up. In that case, she will confront the problem of deciding what to do with the information. In our case, the information was inappropriately learned, while in the case of remembered information, it would only have been recalled.

In any event, now that the counselor knows the information, what should she do with it? In the research setting, it is usually unethical to publish unethically obtained data. However, the question here is harder to resolve. A major (often, the primary) beneficiary of publishing research is the author. One hopes that society or at least the quest for truth also will benefit, but usually the benefits to anyone other than the author are intangible and hard to measure. Therefore, denying publication of unethically obtained data imposes a sanction on the correct person, the ethical transgressor.

Here, however, a real patient and his wife will be the primary beneficiaries of the use of the information. They have not committed any ethical transgression. Moreover, withholding the information from them will result in the wife's undergoing an unnecessary medical procedure that involves some risk to the fetus. Furthermore, they seek prenatal exclusion testing. Because Scott does not want to learn his own risk, we can expect a requested amniocentesis with every pregnancy. Is it appropriate to withhold the benefits of this information—whether remembered or inadvertently obtained—from them?

If there had been no ethical lapse, no information would be available for Scott and his wife. Moreover, they voluntarily sought nondisclosing prenatal testing with whatever risks the procedure entails. To disclose the information now because they could benefit from it adopts a view of ethics that is too narrow because it considers only one set of interests. People are not entitled to every possible benefit just because they are not wrongdoers.

In addition to thinking about Scott and his wife, we should consider the case from the point of view of the couple's relatives and future genetic counselors. To provide this information to these people is to misuse their relatives. The couple can accomplish their goals without that misuse, and their risk in doing so is relatively small. Therefore, disclosure is not justified.

In addition, this result may have some salutary effect in reinforcing the ethical ban on checking the information in the first place. There would be no point in obtaining information that one cannot use. This conclusion is consistent with our refusal to use the sample from the unconsenting aunt after her death in Case 27, "Aunt Mary."

If the counselor had simply remembered the pedigree and linkage information, there would be no future conduct to try to deter. Nonetheless, the information should not be revealed out of respect for commitments made to other family members.

This case is further complicated by the fact that disclosure of the linkage findings would reveal that the patient is not the child of the person he believes to be his father. Revelation of nonpaternity may or may not injure the putative father, depending on how far his dementia has progressed. It is likely to be harmful to Scott's mother; for Scott himself it may be bittersweet, liberating yet opening new issues of concern.

If knowledge of nonpaternity had been gained appropriately, it might well be right to press Scott's mother (if she is living and if she is also a consultand) to explain the situation to her son. We justify comparable advising in Case 7, "Robert," in which a father refuses to inform his daughters of their risk for ADPKD. If Scott's mother is no longer living, or if she remains adamant in denial or refusal to disclose, a breach of confidentiality might be justified to inform Scott of the nonpaternity. However, that conclusion is controversial and represents a close ethical call. The information was not legitimately obtained. Consent for clinical use was never given, and it is entirely possible that no research information would have been obtained if the subjects had known of possible clinical application. Except in extraordinary circumstances, the counselor should not disclose nonpaternity.

Case 29 Mrs. Sawyer

Mrs. Sawyer is a sixty-one-year-old woman at risk for HD; she has not pursued presymptomatic testing for herself and does not plan to do so. She agrees to participate in a research project examining multifactorial genetic influences of the disease. In the course of her daylong participation in the project, Mrs. Sawyer reports that she is in the process of obtaining her pilot's license and flew to the research site from an adjoining state with her flight instructor. As she chats with the research staff, she also reveals that she has yearly physical examinations with her family physician and regularly has been cleared for flying. She also expresses relief that given the fact that the affected members of her family developed symptoms around the age of forty, she is sure that she has "escaped" and will never develop the disease.

In the course of her neurological examination, which is a standard part of the research protocol, the neurologist discovers that Mrs. Sawyer is clearly showing symptoms of HD. The neurologist is concerned about Mrs. Sawyer. She feels that Mrs. Sawyer should not be flying and that if she were to obtain her pilot's license and to fly solo, the results could be disastrous.

The neurologist is aware that all study participants have been assured that they will receive no information regarding their condition. However, she feels that despite the protocol, Mrs. Sawyer should be informed of the results of her neurological examination. Further, she wants to offer to refer her to a neurologist specializing in HD who is closer to her home. Mrs. Sawyer is convinced that she has escaped the disease and is in no way prepared for hearing any information to the contrary. The neurologist fears that giving her this information might upset her so much that she will be unable to fly home. What should the neurologist do?

The core issue raised by this case is a trade-off between commitments the research team made to Mrs. Sawyer as a condition for her entering the protocol (particularly a commitment that she was not to be informed about the results of neurological or genetic testing for HD) and concerns for the public safety raised by her plans to train as a private pilot.

The case differs from Case 11, "Maurice," in two respects. Case 11 raised the issue of breaking promises of confidentiality made to a patient; in the present case, the issue is whether to disclose information to a research subject. Second, Maurice is presymptomatic, whereas Mrs. Sawyer is showing symptoms of HD that are clearly discernible on neurological examination. Thus, it is arguable that the threat to innocent third parties is more immediate in this case.

Mrs. Sawyer agreed to participate in research with the expectation that she would learn nothing about herself, that information would not be forced upon her. The research protocol promised to respect her wish not to seek a diagnosis. Instead, an unwelcome reality is discovered. The obligation to respect her choice not to learn her genetic status is the result of a promise to her; in that respect, it shares a basis with an argument for protecting her confidentiality. Both promises were made to her as conditions of participation in the study.

In this situation, breaking the promise relates to the degree of risk. While Mrs. Sawyer's return flight may present dangers, it is not obvious that they are greater than those posed by other research participants who chose not to learn their risk and who continue to drive automobiles. Both driving and flying might be said to pose serious risks to public safety; neither might; or we might categorically say that the line between driving and flying is a kind of practical benchmark. It seems to us that the neurologist and colleagues at the research site must evaluate the degree of risk on a case-by-case basis. On the facts as presented, it appears that they are justified in breaking their promise to ensure that Mrs. Sawyer does not endanger her own life or the lives of others.

We do not entirely agree about what Mrs. Sawyer should be told. For some of us, her preferences are best respected by generalization and indirection. For example: "You have signs of a movement disorder, and that means it is problematical for you to fly." The explanation could perhaps go on to "and you would be well advised to continue to have regular neurological examinations." The trouble with this euphemistic response is that Mrs. Sawyer is virtually certain to see through it, and its vagueness may be singularly frightening. Thus, our majority feels that it is necessary to tell Mrs. Sawyer the truth: that this neurologist thinks she has discovered symptoms of HD during the examination. This diagnosis need not be presented as final and irrevocable, but it is important that HD be mentioned. Counseling should be offered on the spot, and resources for further counseling or neurological testing should be identified for Mrs. Sawyer.

Obviously this option is only acceptable if the neurologist is sure of her diagnosis. If the diagnosis were uncertain, or if there were alternative ways of protecting others, we would have a different case.

The ultimate point is that research centers should not make promises to subjects that they cannot keep. Mrs. Sawyer's situation is not hard to anticipate. Blanket promises not to inform research participants of findings should only be made with great care, if at all. Once made, however, they should be broken only in rare circumstances.

Guidelines and Commentary

In the following section of the book, we present the guidelines extrapolated from our case analyses. Most of the guidelines are accompanied by a brief commentary that offers an explication, a description of our rationale, and a summary of dissenting positions, if any. In a few instances, specific guidelines seemed to be self-explanatory; they appear without that supplementary material.

Guideline I
Skilled Professional Counseling

I.   The primary obligation of a genetic counselor is to provide skilled professional counseling.

As our cases show, genetic testing will disclose information about individuals seeking testing that those individuals may or may not want to know. A test may generate knowledge that members of consultands' families may want to have or avoid having. Consultands may be making decisions about reproduction, estate planning, organ donation, or other significant life choices. Parents may wish to have their children tested; adult children may wonder about testing incompetent parents. Many of the counselor's consultands are frightened and some are ill-informed. In all of these settings, we have found ourselves concluding that counselors must be more than conduits of information; they should be in the business of giving advice, as the origins of the word *counselor* suggest. In this first guideline, we want to sketch the general parameters of a counselor's role. We want to be as clear as we can about what it means to think of the counselor as an adviser, and what it does not mean. The remaining guidelines will explicate these general ideas.

A.   Counselors should meet with consultands in person. Telephone and mail contact should supplement, not replace, face-to-face communication.

We live in an era when electronic communication is increasingly common, and we can expect these methods of communication to grow in power and accessibility. But we find it difficult to imagine a counseling situation in which communication at a distance is a *sufficient* mode of communication. Some person-to-person contact is necessary. We discuss several cases in which consultands are unwilling to conform to established testing protocols (Cases 21, "Doug"; 23, "Emily"; 24, "Mrs. K."; and 26, "Jackie"), and we will return to that topic. Whatever protocol accommodations may be justified in particular cases, however, we believe that a personal interview should be a component of all genetic counseling.

B. Counselors should devote the time necessary to familiarize themselves with consultands' general health, family, social, psychological, employment, and cultural contexts as well as their genetic condition.

To advise persons about their responsibilities and prospects is a challenging task, especially when one bears in mind the range of issues that may come up. No one person could possibly be expert on the entire range of relevant material, and we discuss the importance of the idea of a counseling team in Guideline III.

In its code of ethics, the National Society of Genetic Counselors emphasizes members' responsibilities to acquire all information necessary to provide competent professional services, to keep current with changing standards of practice, to pursue continued training and education, and to acknowledge the limits of their competence. The code emphasizes values of competence, integrity, dignity, and self-respect and stresses the fundamental importance of care and respect for the consultand's autonomy and welfare (National Society of Genetic Counselors 1992).

C. Counselors should provide information in clear, nontechnical language that is tailored to the intellectual and educational level of the person with whom they are speaking.

Information is useless if it is incomprehensible or misunderstood. Skilled professionals, familiar with the concepts of their field, easily forget just how difficult and confusing specialized terminology may appear to others, particularly to consultands whose knowledge of genetics may be partial, wrong, or misinformed and who may be frightened and worried. Simply presenting a lot of technical information, no matter how correct and precise, is not enough. Counselors must develop the skills to communicate effectively with a wide range of consultands.

When we stress effective communication, we do not wish to prejudge what specific information or what level of detail the consultand will find important and helpful. A first step in effective communication is listening to determine just what the consultand wants to know. The practical implication is that effective communication takes time, as a consultand's need for knowledge may grow and change over time and the counselor must determine that the consultand grasps the essential parts of the complex information presented.

D. Professional counseling requires that counselors go beyond the mere neutral presentation of factual information.

1. Information about diseases, risks, carrier status, treatments, options, and implications must be presented accurately.

2. Information should be presented patiently, tactfully, gently, and with concern for the consultand's well-being.

3. Except in rare circumstances, the counselor should present all relevant information learned in a test to the consultand.

In this guideline we are discussing the issue of withholding *information* acquired in the course of a legitimate testing procedure. The decision of *whether to test* is another matter, one we discuss in Guideline VI. Once a decision to test has been made, however, we find ourselves pushed to a nearly exceptionless rule that the information acquired should be communicated to the consultand. The burden of proof must be on a decision to withhold information, and our cases contain no instances in which that burden can be borne.

A counselor would be far more likely to consider withholding or postponing *testing* than withholding or postponing disclosure of results *after* testing has been completed; the latter course would be highly unusual. The whole point of pretest counseling is to ascertain that the consultand is informed about presymptomatic testing and its implications. Testing protocols include both psychological screening designed to ensure that consultands are emotionally stable, and counseling sessions that help consultands prepare to learn their genetic status. (See Guideline IV.) Hypothetically, test results might be temporarily withheld from a consultand who had experienced a profound personal experience, such as the death of a close family member, in the interval between testing and disclosure. The delay in disclosure would be designed to allow the consultand to regain emotional equilibrium.

a. Withholding test results is justified only when specific, articulable information supports the counselor's professional judgment that receiving the result will lead a particular consultand to make an irrevocable choice of great consequence, such as taking his or her own life.

We believe that this exception would apply in a very small number of cases. Information that justifies withholding results must be *specific*, *articulable*, and the basis of a *professional judgment* rather than an intuition on the counselor's part. The consultand must have explicitly mentioned the possibility of suicide or other irrevocable action, but such a mention is in itself an insufficient justification. Some members of our group believe that a variety of potential adverse outcomes may justify withholding results, including not only threats of suicide but precipitous commitment to or withdrawal from a relationship, or quitting school or a job.

> b. A counselor who has withheld test results for the reason stated in paragraph (a), above, should strive to prepare the consultand to receive full information as soon as possible, and should make full disclosure as soon as doing so is no longer contraindicated on the basis of professional judgment.

We regard a decision to withhold full disclosure as provisional, contingent on the consultand's circumstances at a given time. To the extent possible, the counselor should help consultands prepare themselves so that the information they originally sought can be responsibly transmitted. The counselor may need to refer the consultand to appropriate therapists for assistance. (See the remainder of this Guideline and accompanying commentary.)

> 4. Counselors should not impose their opinions or preferences upon consultands. However, good counseling practice requires counselors to ensure that consultands understand the implications of their decisions for themselves and others, and it may require counselors to offer opinions within the range of their professional expertise.

It is not obvious that genetic counselors should do more than present information. The "workplace ideology" of genetic counseling stresses the ideal of nondirectiveness (Bosk 1992). There are good reasons for this historic emphasis within the profession, including concerns about abuse of power, awareness of the unsavory history of eugenic social policies in the United States and elsewhere, and recognition of the importance of respect for the particular needs and values of individual persons, especially persons who are threatened or unwell.

However, several commentators have argued that it is impossible for genetic counseling to be value-neutral (e.g., Clarke 1991), and we agree. The information provided by genetic testing is highly emotionally charged. Counselors must help consultands by answering questions and providing information to enable them to make informed and reasonable decisions. Counselors should not pretend to have no values or commitments of their own, nor should they fail to share relevant professional experience.

    a.   **The consultand is entitled to the benefit of the counselor's professional expertise. To refuse to share professional insights in the name of "nondirective counseling" is to limit the counselor's usefulness and to provide less than optimal assistance to the consultand.**

We envision counselors and consultands discussing responsibilities to biological family members, spouses, employers, and others affected by the consultands' health, behavior, and sense of self. We do not envision counselors telling consultands *what* they should do in response to their test results. Rather, we argue that counselors must direct consultands to issues and relationships that must be addressed. The counselor need not simply accept the consultands' agenda; rather, the counselor must help consultands to explore their responses to disclosure and to consider the emotional and financial implications of positive or negative test results for themselves and others.

    b.   **Counselors should not share opinions that do not reflect professional expertise.**

We believe that counselors have an obligation to offer consultands the full benefit of their professional expertise. That is why we reject the traditional insistence on nondirective counseling. Nonetheless, we understand the legitimate concerns that lead to a preference for nondirectiveness. The goal of genetic counseling should be to maximize the benefits and minimize the risks of genetic counseling while treating consultands with respect. That is best done by attempting to distinguish matters of professional expertise from those that are not and limiting advice to the former.

It is extremely difficult to distinguish matters of professional expertise. It may be impossible to draw the line in some cases. Every professional person's professional views will be informed by and reflect his or her personal values. Nonetheless, it is important to try to make the distinction and to rule at least clear cases of personal, as opposed to professional, opinions out of bounds.

We take professional expertise to include genetics, other forms of medicine, psychology, counseling skills, and other matters about which the counselor has received formal training in the course of qualifying for a career in genetics or through continuing education programs. Expertise may also include knowledge gained from on-the-job experience, such as awareness of the community resources available to deal with genetic diseases and the problems they present, or the professional's observations of the effect on individuals and families of decisions about such issues as testing and disclosing information. All of these matters may properly inform the professional's judgment and may appropriately be shared with consultands. We offer several suggestions about forms of professional advice that counselors may offer throughout these cases and guidelines. For example, we argue that it is appropriate for counselors to discourage someone from being tested at a particular time, or to advise consultands that they must share information with others in certain instances.

On the other hand, advice that is not rooted in professional education or experience should not be included in the counseling process, either explicitly or implicitly. For example, it would be inappropriate for counselors to base recommendations about prenatal exclusion testing on their own convictions about abortion, whether or not they are rooted in an established religious tradition, or to recommend testing because they believe that everyone must learn his or her exact risk. It is inappropriate for counselors to base recommendations about consultands' behavior on the counselors' nonprofessional beliefs about the consultand's legal position. In other words, genetic professionals should offer professional advice *only* about matters on which they have professional expertise.

Guideline II

Appropriate Information

II.   Professionals should consider ethical issues from the inception of every testing, counseling, and research program, and they should provide consultands with information that is appropriately tailored to the stage of the testing-counseling program the consultand has reached. To the extent possible, ethical dilemmas should be anticipated, and the counselor should try to prevent them from arising.

Our cases repeatedly show instances in which ethical problems arose that might have been avoided with foresight. (See Cases 4, "Ann and Jack"; 8, "Mr. H."; 29, "Mrs. Sawyer.") Reflection on ethical issues should be a part of continuing education for genetic counselors, researchers, and clinicians in genetics. For example, decisions about whether to inform a family member should be considered prior to testing. Foresight and planning can significantly reduce the number of ethical dilemmas that confront counselors. On the whole, it is better to avoid an ethical dilemma, if possible.

A.   Counselors should anticipate the full range of possible findings and test results and their implications and should be prepared in advance to deal with them.

Our cases suggest several areas where anticipation is useful. For example, decisions about whether and what to tell other family members about test results might best be made during pretest counseling. (See Cases 8, "Mr. H," and 9, "Natalie.") Testing centers have been urged to develop policies concerning nonpaternity and to inform consultands about these policies prior to testing (Quaid 1992).

B.   To the extent feasible, counselors should inform consultands in advance about the full range of possible findings, including nonpaternity and diagnoses of mutations or diseases other than those being sought. Counselor and consult-

137

and should reach agreement about how such information and totally unforeseen information will be handled.

At the beginning of the counseling process, the counselor should explain to the consultand the extent to which the process they are beginning is open-ended. Consultands must realize that unwelcome information may become available, and they should have the discretion to broaden or narrow the range of information they will receive. (See Cases 3, "Sarah"; 4, "Ann and Jack"; 8, "Mr. H."; 9, "Natalie"; and 28, "Scott.")

> C. As part of the process of informed consent for genetic research, researchers should discuss with subjects the possibility that research information may become clinically useful and should reach agreement with the subjects about what is to be done if that happens.

We discuss some of the issues arising at the interface between research and clinical application in Guideline IX and the cases cited there. These ambiguities, including the possibility of adventitious findings and changed diagnoses with advances in testing technology, should be explained to the consultand. To the extent that these findings can be anticipated, counselor and consultand should agree in advance on the terms for disclosure.

Guideline III
Pre- and Posttest Counseling

III. Genetic testing should be accompanied by both pre- and posttest counseling conducted by persons with competencies in medical genetics, laboratory analysis, counseling, and the psychosocial impact of genetic information.

It is clear that genetic information is powerful both because the information conveyed is relevant to many decisions and many persons and because it is emotionally charged, with close connection to a consultand's sense of self. This information should not be provided apart from a context in which accuracy and support can be assumed.

We mean to recommend skills that a counselor or—more likely—a counseling team must have. Our list of competencies is meant to illustrate the range of matters counselors may have to discuss with consultands. In correlating these competencies with persons, two errors are possible. One possible inference from Guideline III is that quality counseling can be performed only in a large tertiary care center. We resist that inference. Responsible persons in smaller institutional settings, or well-informed and sensitive solo practitioners, may be able to provide competent counseling on a range of topics, particularly when they refer consultands appropriately to other professionals. On the other hand, we are concerned about ill-informed genetic counseling that may be offered by physicians, nurses, or other health care professionals who are not well acquainted with the particular problems raised by genetic testing and disease.

A. One purpose of counseling *before* testing is to inform the consultand of the risks and benefits of testing and the alternatives to testing, in order to enable the consultand to decide whether or not to be tested and to ensure that the consultand's consent will be voluntary and informed.

Pretest counseling relates directly to processes of securing informed consent, and the counselor must determine whether consent is free and informed. We argue that a formal declaration of incompetence is not always a prerequisite to refusing or postponing testing (Cases 19, "Julie," and 20, "Barbara").

> 1. Consultands *must* be informed about psychological risks and benefits, including impacts on family relationships, as well as physical risks and benefits.

In order to make a truly informed choice, consultands must be informed of certain risks and benefits, just as they must be informed of the risks and benefits of more conventional medical procedures. Consultands who are considering testing must take into account risks to psychological well-being and family relationships, and implications for major life choices.

> 2. Consultands *may* be informed about risks related to employment, insurance coverage, and the possibility of discrimination.

We do not deny the importance of this range of issues, but we can imagine circumstances in which they might not be stressed. On the other hand, they are of such obvious relevance that counselors may well feel that they should mention them in most if not all cases. The crucial point is to provide each consultand with enough information to enable an informed decision about whether to enter the testing process but not to raise issues that may be irrelevant.

> B. Counseling after testing has been performed is designed to help the consultand understand and respond to the test results.

After testing, the counselor's role changes to one of supporting the consultand and assisting him or her in coming to terms with the test results. We believe that this function is extremely important, but it is clear that the consultand may reject the offer of assistance. Posttest counseling cannot be mandated, only recommended, but it can be made available on attractive terms, and it is often a crucial part of responsible transmission of genetic information.

> C. Members of a counseling team should be aware of the limits of their expertise and should refer consultands to persons with relevant specialized knowledge whenever the specialized knowledge is important to the care or counseling of the consultand.

Competent, ethical presymptomatic diagnosis programs must be conducted by teams of professionals who make liberal use of referrals. All responsible counselors will find themselves regularly confronting situations when persons with diverse specialized expertise must be brought into the process. Psychiatric consultation may be crucial in deciding whether to delay or withhold testing; consultation with social workers or other persons informed about the nonmedical effects of genetic disease and carrier status—including lay support groups—can be essential to the consultand's overall well-being; consultands may be referred for appropriate therapy to support them in coming to terms with the implications of their diagnosis. Case 20, "Barbara," presents the problem of appraising the decision-making ability of a consultand who has some mental impairment. The counselor should consult professional colleagues who are experienced in working with such consultands.

D.   Lines of authority within the counseling team must be clearly articulated.

Each team must have a process by which it can resolve differences of opinion and which will ensure that the information given to consultands is clear and coherent. We do not specify what that process must be, but the locus of authority to make decisions must be specified. A good process will ensure that consultands do not receive conflicting or confusing information and will maximize the likelihood that the information they receive represents the team's best thinking.

Guideline IV
Protocols

IV. Protocols are useful guidelines for the appropriate conduct of presymptomatic testing. Justifications for departure from a protocol must relate to the rationale for that protocol.

In this guideline we make some suggestions about the nature, content, firmness, and rationale for genetic testing protocols.

  A. Protocol provisions are rules for counseling procedures and practices that should be related to consultands' medical, psychological, and social needs.

Genetic testing protocols should be grounded in the best interests and integrity of consultands. It is not appropriate to trade off those legitimate interests against either research needs or the convenience of the testing team. While research needs and convenience are relevant and important, neither outweighs consultands' best interests. We do not recommend a specific process for protocol formulation; that issue is outside the scope of our work.

  B. Counselors may depart from or modify protocol provisions only when they have determined that the provisions do not serve the needs of the consultand. Departures from protocol should occur only with team approval.

We do not object to exceptions to testing protocols, if it is clear that the rationale for an exception is consistent with the appropriate rationale for the protocol: serving the interests of the consultand. We endorse departures from protocol in three cases. In Case 21, "Doug," we insisted that psychiatric assessment was essential for a consultand with a stormy history, but we approved flexible arrangements to ensure that he established adequate psychological support. In Case 23, "Emily," we argued that the counselor should explore the consultand's understanding and her reasons for testing. Once satisfied on those points, however, testing could proceed with or without a testing partner. Finally, in Case 24, "Mrs. K.," the consultand was well informed about HD; we agreed that her counseling sessions could be abbreviated to accommodate her level of knowledge.

In Guideline III we discussed the importance of teamwork in a counseling clinic. The present discussion implies that individual counselors are not free to depart from protocol whenever they may choose but must secure the team's agreement, using whatever procedures the team may have established.

    C.   **Counselors should not depart from protocol provisions that they believe are in a consultand's best interests.**

        1.   **Consultand request is not a sufficient basis for departing from protocol provisions.**

A consultand may demand a test immediately (Cases 21, "Doug," and 24, "Mrs. K") or when upset, or may insist on contacting the counselor in unconventional ways (Cases 23, "Emily," and 26, "Jackie"). Family members may demand testing of incompetent, seriously impaired persons or the dead (Case 27, "Aunt Mary"). Although a testing center should be flexible and should respond to consultands' preferences to the extent feasible, testing should only be offered after the counselor is satisfied that it is in the consultand's best interest. (See Guideline I.)

        2.   **Professionals should refuse to follow practices requested by consultands or others that will compromise the professional nature of the practitioner-consultand relationship.**

Important as it is for counselors and counseling to be oriented to the needs of consultands, reasonable procedures must be established to protect counselors' privacy and ability to perform their duties. A counselor contacted away from the workplace, or in irregular ways and times, is unlikely to be able consistently to provide competent counsel. We confront these issues in Case 26, "Jackie," where we resist unusual counseling practices, and Case 23, "Emily," where we tentatively approve them.

Guideline V
Confidentiality

V.   Genetic counselors are ethically obligated to maintain consultands' confidentiality.

Our discussions and guidelines consistently assume the importance of maintaining confidentiality to encourage utilization of services and to respect the dignity and privacy of persons. The consultand shares sensitive information with professionals in exchange for an implicit promise of confidentiality, and that promise should be kept.

The obligation to preserve confidentiality may sometimes be overridden by real and demonstrable needs of public safety, by pressing health needs of the consultands' relatives, and by others' right to make informed decisions.

The obligation to protect confidentiality does not include an obligation—nor does it imply that it is appropriate—to mislead others or to advise the consultand about how to do so.

A.   In general, counselors should not disclose information about consultands or information that is learned from consultands to other persons.

1.   The information that is to be kept confidential includes everything learned from oral and written communication, observation, examination, genetic tests, and all other diagnostic procedures.

We mean to make clear that the obligation of confidentiality applies not only to information disclosed to the counselor but also to the counselor's observations in professional interactions as well as the results of tests of any kind. Occasionally a counselor may have information about a consultand that is a matter of public record, either because they are members of the same community or because the consultand is a public figure. The counselor cannot be expected to keep public information secret but has a normal responsibility not to gossip about the consultand.

144

2.   Counselors and other members of a clinic or testing staff may disclose information about consultands or information that is learned from consultands to other professionals whom the consultand knows are involved in the genetic diagnosis and counseling process and who need the information to contribute to the diagnosis or care of the consultand.

This guideline relates to our preference for genetic counseling to be provided by a team that includes professionals with relevant expertise. (See Guideline III.) Consultands have the right to assume that the information they provide to counselors or other professionals will be confidential. Consultands should be told who is going to have information about them and for what purposes. It is preferable to obtain consultands' permission prior to releasing information even to professionals involved in their care.

Case 5, "Carol," raises the issue of whether a counselor should inform a surgeon about the genetic status of a patient who plans to have a prophylactic mastectomy. There is no universal rule that determines whether surgeons should count as part of the team of professionals in whom a consultand confides. What is essential in this case is that the consultand must know who will have access to confidential medical information about her. Pretest counseling should explore the possibility of prophylactic surgery, and Carol should be informed that the surgeon is obligated to consider her genetic status in weighing the appropriateness of the procedure. Charting and other record-keeping procedures should reflect the confidentiality commitments that have been made to patients.

B.   Confidentiality may be breached when doing so is necessary to protect public safety.

1.   This exception is only applicable when the needs of public safety are real, pressing, and demonstrable.

We deal with this issue in Case 11, "Maurice," when we argue that confidentiality may be breached in the case of someone whose actions may put the lives of thousands of persons at risk. We are more equivocal in Case 29, "Mrs. Sawyer," where the magnitude of the risk is less and the counseling circumstances differ. Throughout our discussion, we intend this exception to apply only in situations in which the needs of public safety are clear and immediate. Everything possible should be done to find a way both to protect the public safety and respect the confidentiality promised to the consultand. Note that in Mrs. Sawyer's case, this requirement explicitly includes respect for a promise that she would not be informed of the results of her examination. This promise to her, like the promise not to disclose test results or examination findings to third parties, may be overridden, but we mean to limit stringently the circumstances in which it may be overridden.

2. The counselor should work with the consultand to attempt to devise a way to protect public safety without breaching confidentiality. Confidentiality may be breached in an emergency or if efforts to work with the consultand have failed.

The counselor should ensure that the consultand grasps the difficulties that failure or refusal to disclose creates for others. The counselor must establish a relationship in which the consultand trusts enough to discuss these kinds of issues, which, among other things, means a relationship in which confidentiality is secure. The counselor should work with the consultand to devise ways in which both the consultand's concerns and others' need to know are respected. If a consultand's adamant refusal to disclose threatens public safety, the counselor may breach confidentiality.

C. In rare instances, a counselor may breach confidentiality in order to serve pressing health needs of a consultand's relatives if doing so will not subject the consultand to unreasonable pressure to submit to risky or invasive procedures.

1. Confidentiality may be breached if providing otherwise confidential information to a relative of the consultand will permit the relative to seek diagnosis or treatment of a serious condition for him- or herself or for someone for whom he or she is responsible.

In considering breaching confidentiality, the counselor should distinguish situations in which other family members know themselves to be at risk from situations in which they are unaware of their risk. It is easier to justify breaching confidentiality for an unsuspecting person than in a situation when risk is being refined.

In Case 7, "Robert," we argue that the consultand is morally obligated to inform his adult daughters that they are at risk for ADPKD. His obligation is more compelling if his daughters are unaware of the family history of the disorder. We conclude that the counselor should try to convince Robert to inform his daughters, and our majority would breach confidentiality if he refuses.

In Case 10, "Mary Ann," a daughter who has been found to carry the BRCA1 gene asks that her test results not be disclosed to her mother, Evelyn, whom she describes as emotionally unstable. We do not recommend breaching confidentiality in that case. Our position is based on the understanding that Evelyn may already be informed of her high risk of breast cancer based on her extensive family history of the disease. Disclosure of Mary Ann's test results may refine Evelyn's risk, but Evelyn can be encouraged to seek adequate health care monitoring without disclosure of Mary Ann's status.

> 2.   **Confidentiality should not be breached if the breach is likely to lead to the consultand being subjected to pressure to imperil his or her own health or to submit to unwanted, invasive medical or surgical procedures such as organ donation.**

In Case 22, "Uncle Lee," a young man has been tested for ADPKD to determine his suitability as an organ donor. His ambivalence about donation to his uncle is clear, as is the fact that he will be under great pressure to donate. Even if we concede that his uncle's need for the kidney is an immediate health need, the uncle's need is outweighed by considerations of the consultand's own health. Donating a kidney is not a risk-free proposition. We do not mean to justify breaching confidentiality if the result is great pressure to run serious medical risks.

> D.   **Counselors should not breach confidentiality to inform consultands' employers or potential employers about a consultand's genetic status except in circumstances as outlined in Guideline VB1 (public safety).**
>
> > 1.   **If a consultand's employer or potential employer asks about the consultand's genetic status, the counselor should refuse to provide the requested information unless the consultand has consented to the disclosure.**
> >
> > 2.   **The counselor should not provide false or misleading information to the employer or potential employer.**

If the consultand has not authorized a release of information, the counselor should simply report that fact. While the counselor has an obligation to protect confidentiality, he or she has no obligation to assist in deceit.

> > 3.   **The counselor should not advise the consultand to**

provide false or misleading information to an employer or potential employer.

The counselor may advise prospective consultands about the possible risks of being tested, including the possibility of genetic discrimination. However, we do not endorse a strategy of helping consultands to deceive present or future employers.

E. If a consultand has applied for health or life insurance and has authorized the disclosure of information to the insurance company, a counselor should answer the insurance company's questions honestly and should make no effort to mislead the company.

1. The counselor has no obligation to volunteer unrequested information to an insurance company.

While the counselor has an obligation to answer all questions honestly and fully, that entails no obligation to guess about other information that the company may find relevant. Volunteering genetic information that has not been requested amounts to a breach of confidentiality.

2. The counselor should not suggest that consultands adopt strategies designed to mislead insurance companies. However, the counselor may answer the consultand's questions about the consequences of the consultand adopting various courses of conduct.

As we explain in Case 12, "Mr. L.," the counselor should discuss the implications of testing with the consultand, including the possibility that insurance coverage may be denied or may be more costly as a result of genetic testing. The counselor should freely respond to the consultand's requests for factual information. However, we do not think that the counselor should assist the consultand in deceiving the insurance company or coach the consultand in equivocation. Counselors should bear in mind that they are probably not experts on insurance.

Guideline VI
Refusing or Postponing Testing

VI. In deciding whether to refuse or postpone testing, genetic counselors should exercise professional judgment based on clinical observation and the consultand's history.

    A.   Testing should usually be provided to adults who seek it. Refusal or postponement should be considered only in exceptional circumstances.

Social resources have been committed to scientific research in genetics; public and private decisions have been made to support genetic testing as a legitimate social activity, including major investments of public funds through the Human Genome Initiative. In these circumstances, the burden of proof must be on a decision to refuse or postpone testing. The counselor must have solid grounds for a professional judgment that testing should be refused or postponed, based on the consultand's responses, behavior, or physical circumstances. (See Cases 18, "Mr. and Mrs. B."; 19, "Julie"; 20, "Barbara"; and 21, "Doug.")

    B.   Postponement of testing is usually preferable to refusal of testing. When testing is postponed, the counselor should attempt to remove the impediment so that testing may be provided with as little delay as possible.

Many (but not all) factors that make testing ill-advised may change with time. A definitive refusal of testing is a last resort, justifiable only if the factors that weigh against testing cannot be changed. In Case 19, "Julie," we recommend that the counselor work with the consultand to help her achieve emotional and social stability. Once that goal is realized, testing should proceed.

    C.   Testing may be postponed if the consultand lacks capacity to give voluntary, informed consent to the testing. If incapacity is permanent, testing may be refused.

Our only case of permanent refusal of testing is Case 20, "Barbara," in which the consultand suffers from intellectual impairment that limits her capacity to provide informed consent. In that case, we stress the importance of an accurate assessment of the consultand's capacities. We insist on the legitimacy of determining competence and of concluding that some persons should not be tested at all.

D. Testing may be postponed if the consultand presents a substantial risk of suicide or is suffering from a psychiatric illness that would seriously compromise his or her ability to cope with test results.

Case 19, "Julie," raises the issues that led to this guideline. Julie has not been declared incompetent, nor is it clear that a court would declare her incompetent. She is emotionally troubled, however; her living circumstances present legitimate grounds for concern; and she has engaged in self-destructive behavior in the past. To be sure, receiving a test result that reveals she does not carry the HD mutation might benefit her, but it might not, and—of course—the test might indicate that she carries the HD mutation.

An interesting twist on this issue comes up in Case 21, "Doug," who refuses psychiatric examination to determine his ability to consent. Given Doug's history of attempted suicide and penal incarceration, we argue that psychosocial evaluation is essential before he proceeds with testing.

We support counselors' decisions to defer testing in cases like Julie's and Doug's, so long as the door remains open to testing if the consultand's circumstances improve. Decisions to postpone will inevitably be judgment calls. We believe that counselors must have professional discretion to avoid a course of action they consider highly risky for a consultand.

E. Testing may be postponed if in the counselor's professional judgment the consultand is ambivalent about undergoing testing or is seeking testing in response to undue pressure applied by other persons.

Many of our cases show the difficulties people have in making up their minds about testing. Only a minority of persons at risk elect genetic testing. This ambivalence may be exacerbated when testing is sought for the benefit of a third party—for example, a prospective spouse, a biological relative, or a prospective recipient of organ donation. (See Case 22, "Uncle Lee.") By this guideline we mean to signal that the counselor must be assured that the consultand him- or herself clearly has decided in favor of testing. Serious ambivalence or indications of great social pressure are plausible reasons to defer testing.

Guideline VII
Freedom to Reject Disclosure

VII. Consultands should remain free to reject disclosure of test results and other diagnostic information unless their decision not to know their status poses a significant risk to others.

We agree that, in the vast majority of cases, test results should not be forced on consultands. We spell out some of the specifics in the first four of the more detailed guidelines that follow (A through D) and consider possible exceptions in the fifth (E).

A. A consultand's participation in testing does not commit the consultand to learn the results of a test.

A consultand may agree to testing in order to help out a family member or to participate in a research study (Case 29, "Mrs. Sawyer"). A person may seek testing and have a change of mind before disclosure (Case 3, "Sarah"). An agreement to participate in testing can be separated from a desire to learn test results. Consultands' decisions, including changes of mind, should be respected. (See Case 5, "Carol.")

B. The consultand's authority to refuse to learn test results should not be affected by what the results reveal. It is as improper for a counselor to force supposedly good news upon a consultand as it is to force a consultand to learn bad news.

Case 3, "Sarah," concerns a young woman who is tested but then declines to learn her test results. In this case, the results are good news; it is tempting to make contact with the consultand and inform her. But we resist this inclination, partly because apparently good news may have its own problems and partly as a matter of respecting the consultand's choice. Moreover, if it becomes known that counselors will aggressively pursue persons who have favorable test results, those who are not pursued may infer the worst.

151

C. The possibility that receiving test results will lead to health-promoting behavior is not a sufficient reason to force information about results on a consultand.

1. If a consultand contemplates submitting to invasive medical procedures because of a mistaken understanding of his or her genetic condition, a counselor should strongly urge the consultand to be fully informed before undergoing the proposed procedure.

In Case 5, "Carol," the consultand already knows that she is at risk for breast cancer because of her family history. Her test results will only inform her whether she carries the BRCA1 gene; in that sense, testing amounts to a refinement of risk. (See Guideline V.) Carol's refusal to learn the results of her test should be respected.

Complications may arise, however. If Carol is contemplating surgical procedures of this magnitude, a counselor would be justified in urging her to learn the results of her test before proceeding. That is not to say that the results of the test should be disclosed over Carol's protest, but to claim that she should be strongly encouraged to learn her test results.

2. Health care professionals should not perform invasive procedures on a patient without first learning the patient's accurate diagnosis and determining that the procedure is, in fact, indicated.

The existence of a genetic test has implications for health care professionals as well as for patients. In Case 5, "Carol," we consider a woman at risk for familial breast cancer who has participated in a research project but has chosen not to learn the results of her test. She contemplates bilateral mastectomy and oophorectomy. We cannot imagine a surgeon performing procedures of that magnitude knowing that a genetic test had been done but unaware of the results of that test. Even if testing does not settle the question of the advisability of prophylactic surgery, test results are obviously relevant and should be part of the diagnostic information. If the prospective patient refuses to release the results of the genetic test to the surgeon, that may well be a signal that the patient's desire for surgery should be more fully explored.

D. The fact that a consultand's refusal of test results may be based on an erroneous assessment by the consultand of his

or her risk is not a sufficient reason to force information
about results upon a consultand, even if the consultand's
misperception is based on information previously learned
from genetic testing or counseling.

In Case 4, "Ann and Jack," we consider a brother and sister whose
results from linkage testing were reversed by a direct gene test. When the
old samples were rerun without their knowledge or consent, both siblings tested positive for the HD mutation. The testing center has informed them that new information is available if they want it. The center
has sent them a detailed letter explaining the accuracy of the new testing
procedure and specifically stating that linkage results may be revised and
even reversed. Ann and Jack declined reevaluation. We resist the idea that
they should be exhorted to undergo retesting, even though they have
been nonnegligently misinformed by the center. Although Ann and Jack
once wanted to know their risk, they have declined the opportunity to
have their risk refined. Their decision should be respected.

E.   Unwanted information may be disclosed to a consultand, if
     the counselor determines that without the information the
     consultand is likely to engage in behavior that endangers
     others.

We confront this issue in Case 29, "Mrs. Sawyer." In that case, we
consider a woman who has agreed to participate in a research study. She
has been informed that she will receive no clinical information as a result
of her participation, but on detailed neurological examination she shows
clear symptoms of HD. She flew a private plane to the testing center. *If*
Mrs. Sawyer's symptoms have reached a point where she poses a clear
danger to others (an inference that cannot be drawn with certainty from
the facts of the case), we agree that the counselor must take steps to keep
her from putting other persons at serious risk.

We disagree, however, on the nature of these steps. Some members
of our group argue that Mrs. Sawyer should be informed that she is
showing symptoms of a "movement disorder" in an attempt to plant
seeds of doubt regarding her condition. She could be urged to pursue
diagnosis when she returns home. This course would provide more time
for Mrs. Sawyer. The other faction disagrees, arguing that she should be
informed immediately that she is showing symptoms of HD. This group
believes that candor is the best approach. Mrs. Sawyer will soon learn
that she has HD, so that euphemistic references to a "movement disor-

der" will not serve her best interest. Further, informing her immediately will protect the public, if her symptoms are advanced enough to make that consideration relevant.

In Case 9, "Natalie," we consider the counselor's responsibility to Helen, a sample provider who does not think she is at risk; testing, however, reveals her risk to be significant. We argue that the option of learning her own results should be presented to her, but our reason is related to her choices and interests, not a risk she poses to anyone else.

Guideline VIII
Others' Preference Not to Know

VIII. The fact that testing a consultand will reveal the genetic status of other persons, who prefer not to know their status, is not, by itself, a sufficient reason to delay testing.

Much as we wish to respect someone's choice not to learn his or her own risk of a genetic disorder, that choice does not trump the desire of other persons at risk to learn whether they carry a particular allele of interest. Important as it may be for one individual not to know, that person should not be able to enforce that preference on another. Crucial cases for our discussion of this point are Cases 1, "Paul and Michael"; 2, "Father and Son"; and 6, "Kirsten and David." In each of those cases, the counselor is pressed to withhold testing from one person because of the preferences of another. We argued that the individual seeking testing should be tested, if his or her own psychological profile and other factors indicate that testing is appropriate. Another person's choice not to know alone should not settle the question.

   A. Additional factors that, combined with a second person's choice not to know, might justify a decision to delay testing include:

      1. The closeness of the relationship between the consultand and the other person who may gain unwanted information.

Our cases include very close family relationships—some biological and some not. The case for withholding testing might be weaker if the relationships were more distant (for example, cousins who are not acquainted).

      2. The existence of a professional relationship between the counselor and the other person.

If the person who chooses not to know is also the counselor's consultand, the counselor may feel torn between a duty to maintain confidentiality and a responsibility to provide helpful and desired information to another consultand. It may be useful to bring in a second counselor for one of the parties in such a situation.

> 3. The gravity of the risk to the other person of receiving the unwanted information.

Differing degrees of vulnerability must be taken into account; it matters if unwanted disclosure will lead to mild anxiety or a likelihood of self-destruction.

None of these possibilities is necessarily a reason to withhold testing, but the reasonably predictable consequences for others cannot be dismissed as irrelevant. While we think it unlikely that a constellation of such factors can outweigh a consultand's request for appropriate testing, we do not think it impossible. Other identifiable, living persons may have interests in the consultand's being tested, and these interests cannot be summarily dismissed.

> B. When testing a consultand poses a foreseeable risk of psychological harm to another person, the counselor should discuss the risk with the consultand, explore the consultand's ethical responsibilities, and encourage the consultand to make affirmative efforts to protect the other person from harm.

Whether or not testing is delayed, we think counselors should spend time with consultands going over the range of considerations and interests of others that weigh against testing; the consultand needs to see why her or his choice is problematical for others. We discuss this general point under Guideline I. In our most relevant cases, it is important for Kirsten to see what her insistence on testing is saying to David about him (Case 6), and for Paul to understand why Michael may not want this information (Case 1). Part of the counselor's responsibility is to force consultands to think through issues they may prefer to ignore.

> C. In considering whether to delay testing to avoid informing another person of his or her status, the counselor should not consider alleged interests of "society."

Although we hold that a social decision to establish genetic counseling programs implies that people should have access to genetic information (see Case 6, "Kirsten and David"), we do not wish to draw the inference that broad social utility factors should enter into consideration of whether to test a specific individual. Those decisions should be made on the merits of the case.

D.   Any delay of testing to protect another person should be only long enough to provide counseling and to give the consultand time to absorb and act on it.

We suggest that delays of a matter of weeks, rather than months or years, are appropriate. If testing is delayed to protect another who declines to know his or her genetic status, the delay should be provisional and of distinctly limited duration.

Guideline IX
Possible Future Uses of Information

IX. Persons engaged in clinical genetics and genetic research should discuss with potential subjects the possible future uses of the information acquired. This discussion should be part of the informed consent process for participation in the research. At the time they enter into a research or clinical genetics program, subjects or patients may also give informed consent to future use of information about them.

An individual who is contemplating providing information or a sample for genetic testing or research should know the terms under which the information or material will be used. Those terms may be very broad. Subjects may consent to the use of their blood or tissue samples or information they provide for a range of purposes—purely research-related or clinically significant for the subject or members of the subject's family. Alternatively, the terms governing use of information or samples may be narrow: The subject may consent only to provide information for research purposes or explicitly reject its use for clinical purposes (Cases 5, "Carol"; 29, "Mrs. Sawyer"), or the person may refuse to provide a sample for any purpose whatsoever (Case 27, "Aunt Mary"). The crucial thing is that the terms of the arrangement be clear at the outset and that all parties understand and agree to them.

A. Research specimens collected for a specific research study should not be used for any other purpose or study unless each specimen is completely stripped of all identifiers.

In Case 28, "Scott," a counselor examines an extensive family pedigree to discover that a man requesting prenatal testing is not at risk of HD because of nonpaternity. We argue against using information like this even for clearly good purposes. In that case, the counselor confirmed her memory by checking records; we would hold the same view if the only form of data recall available were the counselor's memory.

158

B. In the case of information clearly restricted to research uses at the time of collection, relevant clinical information should be used only when it is necessary to protect the public safety.

In Case 29, "Mrs. Sawyer," members of a research team debate revealing a diagnosis of HD to a woman who agreed only to participate in a research project. Although she expected to undergo a daylong series of neurological, psychological, and biological tests, a condition of her participation was that clinical information would not be shared with subjects. Some of us think that condition should be honored, even though a stronger case might be made for revealing a clinical diagnosis than the results of a genetic test. It seems to us that a neurological examination conducted as part of a research protocol should lead the researchers to urge that their subject seek additional *clinical* consultation. However, *if* it is clear that informing Mrs. Sawyer is the only way to protect the public safety, we concede that Mrs. Sawyer must be told the results of her neurological examination. To justify this violation of research protocol, the threat to public safety should be clear, significant, and certain.

Others in our group, however, argue that Mrs. Sawyer should be informed of her diagnosis candidly and immediately, for her own sake as well as that of the public.

C. Even if information was originally collected for clinical purposes, it should not be reanalyzed using new and improved tests without the subject's permission. If samples are retested and subjects are given the opportunity to learn the new results, refusal of this opportunity must be respected.

The subjects who participated in a study may be asked if they object to having their samples reanalyzed or used for clinical purposes. In Case 4, "Ann and Jack," we resist any additional use of samples if the technology changes and a new or better test is developed. A parallel issue is raised in Case 9, "Natalie." If a new test becomes available, persons who were originally tested using one method may be notified by the testing center of the improved technology and asked whether they would like to have their tests rerun. The new terms and facts can be explained to them, and they may or may not opt for reanalysis.

A minority of our group feels that it is legitimate to retest a sample if an improved testing technology becomes available. Even in this view, however, the subjects should not be informed of the result of the new test without their consent.

> D. Researchers should anticipate the discovery of clinically relevant information and should design appropriate methods of disclosing that information to participants who request it. Information derived through research projects may be provided to participants only when adequate counseling and support are available.

Case 29, "Mrs. Sawyer," illustrates the problem this Guideline is meant to address. Persons may be willing to participate in a study despite grave reluctance to learn more about their own risk. But circumstances may arise in which it is difficult or morally impossible to keep this knowledge from them. Therefore, testing programs should be prepared to take on counseling responsibilities.

Guideline X
Reproductive Choices

X. Genetic counselors and other professionals should not force reproductive choices onto consultands. However, they should counsel consultands about the full implications of their choices.

We take it as axiomatic that decisions surrounding reproduction are properly the decisions of prospective parents; such decisions are not to be made by the state, advocacy groups, or professionals, including genetic counselors. That said, reproductive choices are consequential, and we do not exclude them from the zone of choices in which counselors may offer well-informed professional advice.

   A. Genetic professionals may not ethically withhold prenatal diagnosis from a pregnant woman because the fetus's father—or some other family member—opposes the testing.

We reach this conclusion in Case 6, "Kirsten and David." In that case Kirsten, who is pregnant, wants prenatal testing. Her husband David, who is at risk for HD, does not want prenatal testing. We argued that the consequences of denying Kirsten the test outweigh the risks to David of performing the test. This guideline simply applies the principle to other family members beyond the individual at risk, who is the biological father of the fetus. We go on to stress the importance of active counseling with Kirsten to ensure that she is aware of the consequences and implications for David of her insistence upon the test. We regard this step as part of the counselor's duty to promote informed reproductive decision making. If, after counseling, the pregnant woman insists on prenatal testing, testing should be performed. The counselor should offer his or her services to David and to the couple in posttest counseling to attempt to minimize any harm to David.

   B. Provision of genetic services should not be provisional upon a commitment to abort fetuses who carry mutations.

When a fetus tests positive for HD and the pregnancy is carried to term, the child will be a known mutation carrier from birth. In this situation, prenatal testing is tantamount to presymptomatic testing of a child.

In Case 18, "Mr. and Mrs. B.," we discuss a genetic testing center's policy that requires a couple seeking prenatal diagnosis to agree to abort fetuses that carry the HD mutation. Our majority agrees with the center's underlying goal—that children should not undergo presymptomatic testing for HD. The testing center wants to signal its opposition to that outcome in the strongest possible terms.

However, we argue that a policy of requiring a commitment to abort is unlikely to be effective; moreover, it suggests a return to the rightly discredited image of the geneticist as eugenicist. The policy is understandable but clumsy, indeed so clumsy as to be morally wrong.

Nevertheless, we think it important for professionals to counsel couples who seek prenatal diagnosis about the undesirability of presymptomatic testing of children for untreatable late-onset genetic conditions. At least in the case of HD, prospective parents need to understand why many knowledgeable and thoughtful persons feel that children should not be tested, and that a decision to test a fetus that will be brought to term irrevocably violates that standard.

Guideline XI
Testing Children

XI. Genetic testing of *symptomatic* children to make or confirm a diagnosis may be performed subject to general ethical and legal rules governing medical care for children. *Presymptomatic* genetic testing should only be performed on children when all of the conditions set out in paragraphs A, B and C are met.

If a child is showing symptoms, and if genetic testing is the only or best way to confirm a diagnosis, genetic testing is appropriate and non-controversial. In contrast, a majority of our group believes there must be restrictions on *presymptomatic* testing of children. We distinguish disorders in which presymptomatic testing confers a medical benefit from those in which it does not, and we argue that few situations exist to justify presymptomatic testing of a child for a late-onset disorder for which little or nothing can be done. We develop our arguments for this conclusion in Cases 13, "Mr. Crawford," and 14, "Mr. and Mrs. Anderson." These cases are driven by the conviction that persons should be able to choose for themselves as adults whether to learn their genetic status.

A minority of our group reserves decision-making authority over presymptomatic testing to the parents even in late-onset disorders for which cure or treatment is not available. They argue that parents are entitled to make other decisions governing their children's medical care; presymptomatic genetic testing does not constitute an exception. Professionals may override parental wishes only on a case-by-case basis when the usual reasons for deference to parents' judgment are lacking.

We do not offer a special definition of "child" or "competence," and we recognize that hard cases will arise, perhaps in the late primary and middle school years. We do not discuss other special legal categories such as "emancipated minors." Our intention is to restrict presymptomatic testing until consultands have reached a level of maturity that ensures they are clearly able to provide informed consent. These hard issues are not unique to the context of genetic testing.

A. **A presymptomatic test should be given to a child only if both of the child's parents who are reasonably available have consented to the testing. If only one parent is reasonably available, that parent must consent to the testing.**[3]

We do not assume that all parents can always be reached or that parents must travel great distances. On the other hand, presymptomatic testing normally will not be considered a true emergency, and hasty conclusions should be avoided in situations with stakes so high. The effect of this guideline is to honor our majority's view of the burden of proof: If parents disagree about testing their child, then the verdict goes to the party who opposes testing. It is the decision to test that is irrevocable. Testing can be done later, when parents or guardians agree or when the child has reached an age to decide for himself or herself. Note that parental consent is not the only relevant criterion.

B. **If the child has or can be provided with a reasonable understanding of the proposed genetic test and its implications, the child's assent to genetic testing must be sought.**

We think that children who understand what is going on should not be tested over their protests. The child will have to live with the results of learning the information. For example, in Case 15, "Jimmy," we are troubled by the fact that an adolescent's own opinion about whether to be tested seems never to have been sought.

This requirement will become controversial in cases where testing offers the possibility of real benefit to the child, but the child nevertheless refuses to be tested. Even then, the child's assent is important. For example, a child at risk for familial adenomatous polyposis might refuse both testing and recommended annual screening sigmoidoscopies. Because regular screening is an adequate way to monitor the child's condition, the child's choice against *testing* should be respected. On the other hand, parental responsibility for regular screening is comparable to parental responsibility for other medical care for children who have reached the age of assent. Some such *screening* procedures may have to be done over the child's protest. If the child were seriously endangered, and if the *only* way to determine the best treatment were presymptomatic testing, the parents might authorize the test over the child's objection. We did not confront such a case.

---

3. The guardian of a child may act in place of a parent.

C.   There must be a reasonable possibility that testing will enable the child to receive a real, demonstrable benefit.

Broadly speaking, we hold that testing must offer the possibility of tangible benefit to the child. Possible sociological, psychological, or economic benefits are insufficient. We specify some factors below.

1.   Some examples of real, demonstrable benefits are: medical treatment and medical monitoring that permits early intervention to cure or alleviate disease.

In Case 16, "Harriet," we favor testing of children at risk for FAP. A negative test will liberate the children from a noxious regimen of surveillance procedures; a positive test will justify medical monitoring and may influence decisions related to medical interventions.

2.   The following do not constitute sufficiently real, demonstrable benefits to the child to justify presymptomatic testing:

a.   relief of the child's or parents' anxiety.

In contrast to Case 16, "Harriet," where genetic testing for FAP will confer a medical benefit, we have two cases in which parents request that their children be tested to relieve parental anxiety. In Case 15, "Jimmy," the mother of a child at risk for ADPKD wants her son tested; in Case 17, "Charley," a mother wants her child tested for HD even though the likely diagnosis is Tourette's syndrome. The adolescent at risk for ADPKD is faithfully following recommended medical screening and will soon be in a position to make his own choice about testing. The child at risk for HD can have a more thorough clinical workup to support a possible diagnosis. Testing offers no immediate medical benefit for these children and risks loss of self-determination. They should not be tested.

b.   parental or other desires to make special financial arrangements, educational plans, or career counseling for children based on their genetic status.

Case 13, "Mr. Crawford," deals with a grandfather who wants to provide appropriately for his grandchildren. He could be more confident about his arrangements if he knew whether his two grandchildren at risk carry the mutation for HD. We concluded that he could attain his ends in other ways and that the grandfather's wishes do not control in decisions about testing the children.

D. Concerns about the presymptomatic testing of children are not sufficient to justify conditioning prenatal testing on parental agreement to abort affected fetuses.

Prenatal testing should not be used as a way of getting around the general prohibition of testing children. When they come of age, children may decide for themselves whether they wish to be tested. But that does not justify manipulative policies on prenatal testing. (See Guideline X.B. and comments.)

Glossary

Allele. One of the alternative or variant sequences of a particular segment of DNA; one form of a given gene.

At risk. Occupying a position in a pedigree at which a genetic mutation may be inherited.

Autosome. Any chromosome other than a sex chromosome (x or y).

Autosomal dominant. A mutation carried on an autosome; a mutation of one allele is sufficient to confer the disease genotype. Each offspring of a parent affected by an autosomal dominant disorder has a 50 percent chance of inheriting the mutation.

Autosomal dominant polycystic kidney disease (ADPKD). One of the most common genetic disorders, affecting more than 500,000 individuals in the United States. ADPKD causes replacement of normal kidney tissue by abnormal fluid-filled cysts, resulting in renal failure.

BRCA1. A gene located on chromosome 17q that when damaged dramatically increases the risk of breast and ovarian cancer.

CAG repeat (see *Trinucleotide repeat*). A repeating pattern of three nucleotide bases (CAG), found in patients with Huntington disease and several other diseases.

Carrier. A person who has at least one mutant allele but is usually asymptomatic for the disorder.

Choreiform. "Dancelike"; a neurological term that refers to involuntary flapping or jerking movements made by individuals with a neurological disorder such as Huntington disease.

Consultand. A person seeking and receiving counseling.

Direct testing. Genetic testing that determines whether an individual has a mutant gene. (See *Linkage testing.*)

Exon. The coding sequence of a gene.

Familial adenomatous polyposis (FAP). An autosomal dominant familial colon cancer syndrome characterized by hundreds of polyps found in the colon. See Introduction.

Fiduciary. In the nature of a trust. A fiduciary relationship is one in which the entrusted person (e.g., health professional) is obligated to act on behalf of another person (e.g., consultand), to put the other's interests first, and to act toward the other with the utmost good faith.

Gene marker. A DNA segment used in genetic studies. DNA markers usually are localized to a chromosome and have distinguishable alleles. (See *Restriction fragment length polymorphism [RFLP]*.)

Genome. The total DNA content of an organism.

Genotype. The genetic composition of an individual. (See *Phenotype*.)

Haplotype. The genetic makeup of a single chromosome or chromosomal region.

Human Genome Project. The federally funded effort to identify polymorphic genetic markers spaced throughout the genome at a high density and to provide physical maps that show the location of functionally expressed genes and their sequences as a basis for the elucidation, and eventual prevention and cure, of human diseases. (See *Science* 256 [April 24, 1992]: 480.)

Huntington disease (HD). An incurable, degenerative neuropsychiatric disease characterized by a choreiform movement disorder, dementia, and affective disturbances. HD is inherited as an autosomal dominant trait with complete lifetime penetrance, so that all who inherit the mutation develop the disease, assuming they survive to the time of symptom onset (usually around age forty). It is caused by a mutation on chromosome 4, a CAG *trinucleotide repeat.*

Linkage analysis. The estimation of the distance between a genetic marker and the gene of interest.

Linkage testing (also see *Direct testing*). A form of genetic testing that identifies the presence of a genetic marker linked to the gene in question. Linkage testing is possible when a genetic marker has been identified but the specific genetic mutation has not yet been "mapped" or defined. It requires DNA samples from family members who are affected and family members who have outlived the age of onset of symptoms in their family but have not developed the disease ("escapees"). DNA from those seeking testing is then compared with these family members' samples to determine whether the testees' DNA matches that of the affected or the unaffected relatives. Because the marker is near the mutation but is not itself the mutation, linkage results may not be completely accurate. Due to the phenomenon of recombination, the chromosomes in a homologous pair may trade segments of DNA during meiosis. Thus, the marker may separate from the gene in question, rendering the results of testing inaccurate for any individual who has inherited a separated gene-marker combination. The likelihood of recombination is proportionally related to the distance between the marker and the gene. (See *Linkage analysis.*)

Negative. A test result that indicates that an individual does not carry the gene mutation tested for.

Nondisclosing prenatal testing. Genetic testing of a fetus that does not reveal the genetic status of the parent at risk. For example, consider the pedigree in

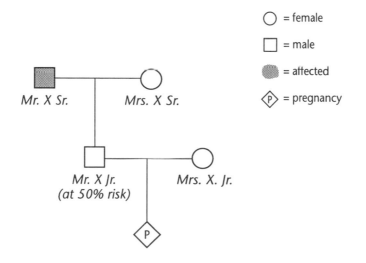

the diagram. In this pedigree, Mr. X., Jr. is at 50 percent risk of inheriting HD, an autosomal dominant disease, from his affected father. He has inherited one chromosome 4 from his affected father and one from his mother, but he does not know whether the chromosome he inherited from his father carries the mutant gene. Now the fetus is tested to determine which Grandparent X. contributed the chromosome 4 that came from its father's side of its family. If the fetus has inherited a chromosome 4 from Grandmother X., it has not inherited the mutant chromosome. If the fetus's chromosome 4 is inherited from Grandfather X., however, it is at 50 percent risk of inheriting HD; its risk is the same as that of its father, Mr. X., Jr. Mr. X., Jr. is not tested, and the test of the fetus reveals no additional information about the genetic status of Mr. X., Jr. Typically, a couple seeking nondisclosing prenatal testing intends to terminate the pregnancy if the fetus has inherited its chromosome 4 from the affected grandparent, despite the 50 percent chance that the fetus has *not* inherited the mutant gene. (See also *Linkage testing.*)

Penetrance. The proportion of individuals who express the phenotype dictated by a specific genotype.

Phenotype. The visible characteristics of an individual. (See *Genotype.*)

Positive. A test result that indicates that an individual carries the gene mutation tested for.

Predictive test. A genetic test that can identify a gene or gene marker. Predictive testing can foretell the development of or predisposition to a certain disease and can provide information about the likelihood that the disease will appear at some time in the future; it currently provides no information about the patient's age at onset of disease or the severity of the illness. "Predictive testing" may refer to *linkage testing* or *direct genetic testing.*

Prenatal exclusion testing. See *Nondisclosing prenatal testing.*

Presymptomatic. Devoid of symptoms of a particular disorder; symptoms may develop in the future.

Presymptomatic test. A test performed on an individual who has no signs or symptoms of the genetic disorder for which the test is being performed.

Proband. The first person in a family who is diagnosed with a particular genetic disorder.

Professional judgment. A value judgment based on values that justify the professional practice (e.g., the provision of counsel), distinguished from judgments based on the commitments or life plans of individual practitioners.

Restriction fragment length polymorphism (RFLP). An allele characterized by variations in the length of DNA fragments cut by a given restriction endonuclease at a given sequence. A restriction endonuclease is a kind of enzyme that cleaves DNA at every site where a specific sequence occurs. For example, the enzyme Alu 1 (from Arthrobacter luteus) recognizes the sequence AGCT and cuts it between G and C. Individuals may vary in the lengths of the DNA fragments that result from these cleavages, and the variable DNA lengths that result can be used as genetic markers.

Trinucleotide. Any combination of three amino acids.

Trinucleotide repeat (see *CAG repeat*). A trinucleotide that appears multiple times within a particular genetic sequence.

Tumor suppressor gene. A gene whose function is to impede or control cellular replication and growth.

References

Adam, S.; Wiggins, S.; Lawson, K.; McKellin, B.; and Hayden, M. R. "Predictive Testing for Huntington Disease (HD): Differences in Uptake and Characteristics of Linked Marker and Direct Test Cohorts." *American Journal of Human Genetics Supplement*, Abstract 1698 57 (1995): A292.

Alper, J. S. "Does the ADA Provide Protection against Discrimination on the Basis of Genotype?" *Journal of Law, Medicine and Ethics* 23 (1995): 167–72.

American Cancer Society. *Cancer Facts and Figures.* Atlanta: American Cancer Society, 1995, pp. 10–11.

The American College of Medical Genetics/American Society of Human Genetics Huntington Disease Genetic Testing Working Group. "ACMG/ASHG Statement on Laboratory Guidelines for Huntington Disease Genetic Testing." *American Journal of Human Genetics* 62 (1998): 1243–47.

The American Society of Human Genetics Board of Directors and The American College of Medical Genetics Board of Directors. "ASHG/ACMG Report. Points to Consider: Ethical, Legal, and Psychosocial Implications of Genetic Testing in Children and Adolescents." *American Journal of Human Genetics* 57 (1995): 1233–41.

Andrew, S. E; Goldberg, Y. P.; Kremer, B.; et al. "The Relationship between Trinucleotide (CAG) Repeat Length and Clinical Features of Huntington's Disease." *Nature Genetics* 4 (1993): 398–403.

Andrews, Lori B.; Fullarton, Jane E.; Holtzmann, Neil A; and Motulsky, Arno G. (Committee on Assessing Genetic Risks, Division of Health Sciences Policy, Institute of Medicine); eds. *Assessing Genetic Risks: Implications for Health and Social Policy*. Washington, D.C.: National Academy Press, 1994.

Arras, John D. "AIDS and Reproductive Decisions: Having Children in Fear and Trembling." *Milbank Quarterly* 68, 3 (1990): 353–82.

Barash, Carol. "At-Risk Persons Report Episodes of Discrimination." *Marker* (Spring 1994): 10.

Bear, J. C. (1995) "ADPKD: Practical Implications of Population Genetics. *Contributions to Nephrology* 115 (1995): 20–27.

Bear, J. C.; McMaraman, P.; Morgan, J.; Payne, R. H.; Lewis, H.; Gault, M. H.; and Churchill, D. N. "Age at Clinical Onset and at Ultrasonographic Detection of Adult Polycystic Kidney Disease: Data for Genetic Counseling." *American Journal of Medical Genetics* 18 (1984): 45–53.

Benjamin, C. M.; Adam, S.; Wiggins, S.; Theilmann, J. L.; Copley, T. T.; Bloch,

M.; Squitieri, F.; McKellin, W.; Cox, S.; Brown, S. A.; Kremer, H. P. H.; Burgess, M.; Meshino, W.; Summers, A.; Macgregor, D.; Buchanan, J.; Greenberg, C.; Carson, N.; Ives, E.; Frecker, M.; Welch, J. P.; Fuller, A.; Rosenblatt, D.; Miller, S.; Dufrasne, S.; Roy, M.; Andermann, E.; Prevost, C.; Khalifa, M.; Girard, K.; Taylor, S.; Hunter A.; Goldsmith, C.; Whelan, D.; Eisenberg, D.; Soltan, H.; Kane, J.; Shokeir, M. H. K.; Gibson, A.; Cardwell, S.; Bamforth, S.; Grover, S.; Suchowersky, O.; Klimek, M.; Garber, T.; Gardner, H. A.; MacLeod, P.; and Hayden, M. R. "Proceed with Care: Direct Predictive Testing for Huntington Disease." *American Journal of Human Genetics* 55 (1994): 606–17.

Billings, Paul R., et al. "Discrimination as a Consequence of Genetic Testing. *American Journal of Human Genetics* 50 (1992): 476–82.

Bloch, Maurice; Adam, Shelin; Wiggins, Sandy; Huggins, Marlene; and Hayden, Michael R. "Predictive Testing for Huntington Disease in Canada: The Experience of Those Receiving an Increased Risk." *American Journal of Medical Genetics* 42 (1992): 499–507.

Bloch, Maurice; Fahy, M.; Fox, S.; and Hayden, Michael R. "Predictive Testing for Huntington Disease: II. Demographic Characteristics, Life-Style Patterns, Attitudes, and Psychosocial Assessments of the First Fifty-One Test Candidates." *American Journal of Medical Genetics* 32 (1989): 217–24.

Bloch, M., and Hayden, M. R. "Predictive Testing for Huntington Disease in Childhood: Challenges and Implications (Opinion)." *American Journal of Human Genetics* 46 (1990): 1–4.

Bosk, Charles L. *All God's Mistakes: Genetic Counseling in a Pediatric Hospital.* Chicago: University of Chicago Press, 1992.

Brandt, Jason; Quaid, Kimberly A.; Folstein, Susan E.; Garber, Paul; Maestri, Nancy E.; Abbott, Margaret H.; Slavney, Phillip R.; Franz, Mary L.; Kasch, Laura; and Kazazian, Haig H., Jr. "Presymptomatic Diagnosis of Delayed-Onset Disease with Linked DNA Markers: The Experience in Huntington's Disease." *Journal of the American Medical Association* 261 (1989): 3108–14.

Bulow, S. "Familial Polyposis Coli." *Danish Medical Bulletin* (1987) 34: 1–15.

Burgess, M., and Hayden, M. R. "Patients' Rights to Laboratory Data: Trinucleotide Repeat Length in Huntington Disease." *American Journal of Medical Genetics* 62 (1996): 6–9.

Caskey, C. T. "II. Presymptomatic Genetic Diagnosis: A Worry for the United States." In George J. Annas and S. Elias, eds., *Gene Mapping Using Law and Ethics as Guides.* New York: Oxford University Press, 1992.

Castilla, L. H.; Couch, F. J.; Erdos, M. R.; et al. "Mutations in the BRCA1 Gene in Families with Early-Onset Breast and Ovarian Cancer." *Nature Genetics* 8 (1994): 387–91.

Chapman, Marguerite A. "Invited Editorial. Canadian Experience with Predictive Testing for Huntington Disease: Lessons for Genetic Testing Centers and Policy Makers." *American Journal of Medical Genetics* 42 (1992): 491–98.

Clarke, Angus. "Is Non-directive Genetic Counselling Possible? *Lancet* 338 (1991): 998–1001.

Clarke, David J., and Bundey, Sarah. "Very Early Onset Huntington's Disease: Genetic Mechanism and Risk to Siblings." *Clinical Genetics* 38 (1990): 180–86.

Clinical Genetics Society (U.K.). "The Genetic Testing of Children." *Journal of Medical Genetics* 31 (1994): 785–97.

Codori, A. M., and Brandt, J. "Psychological Costs and Benefits of Predictive Testing for Huntington Disease." *American Journal of Medical Genetics (Neuropsychiatric Genetics)* 54 (1994): 174–84.

Collins, F. S. "BRCA1—Lots of Mutations, Lots of Dilemmas." *New England Journal of Medicine* 334 (1996): 186–88.

Conneally, P. M. "Huntington Disease: Genetics and Epidemiology." *American Journal of Human Genetics* 36 (1984): 506–36.

Conneally, P. M.; Haines, J. L.; Tanzi, R. E.; Wexler, N. S.; Penchaszadeh, G. K.; Harper, P. S.; Folstein, S. E.; Cassiman, J. J.; Myers, R. H.; Young, A. B.; Hayden, M. R.; Falek, A; Tolosa, E. S.; Crespi, S.; Di Maio, L; Holmgren, G.; Anvret, M.; Kanazawa, I.; and Gusella, J. F. "Huntington Disease: No Evidence for Locus Heterogeneity." *Genomics* 5 (1989): 304–8.

Corson, Virginia; Quaid, Kimberly; Kasch, Laura; and Kazazian, Haig H., Jr. "Prenatal Testing for Huntington Disease." *Birth Defects Original Article Series* 26, 3 (1990): 226–30.

Crandall, B.; Kulch, P.; and Tabsh, K. "Risk Assessment of Amniocentesis between 11 and 15 Weeks: Comparison to Later Amniocentesis Controls." *Prenatal Diagnosis* 14 (1994): 913–19.

Craufurd, D.; Dodge, A; Kerzin-Storrar, L.; and Harris R. "Uptake of Presymptomatic Predictive Testing for Huntington's Disease." *Lancet* (September 9, 1989): 603–5.

Davies, F.; Coles, G. A.; Harper, P. S.; Williams, A. J.; Evans, C.; and Cochlin, D. "Polycystic Kidney Disease Re-evaluated: A Population-based Study." *Quarterly Journal of Medicine* 79 (1991): 477–85.

DeGrazia, David. "The Ethical Justification for Minimal Paternalism in the Use of the Predictive Test for Huntington's Disease." *Journal of Clinical Ethics* 2, 4 (1991): 219–28.

Duyao, M.; Ambrose, C.; Myers, R.; et al. "Trinucleotide Repeat Length Instability and Age of Onset in Huntington's Disease." *Nature Genetics* 4 (1993): 387–92.

Easton, D. F.; Bishop D. T.; Ford, D.; Crockford G. P.; and the Breast Cancer Linkage Consortium. "Genetic Linkage Analysis in Familial Breast and Ovarian Cancer: Results from 214 Families." *American Journal of Human Genetics* 52 (1993): 678–701.

Easton, D. F.; Ford, D.; Bishop, D. T.; and the Breast Cancer Linkage Consortium. "Breast and Ovarian Cancer Incidence in BRCA1-Mutation Carriers." *American Journal of Human Genetics* 56 (1995): 265–71.

Emanuel, Ezekiel J., and Emanuel, Linda L. "Four Models of the Physician-Patient Relationship." *Journal of the American Medical Association* 267 (1992): 2221–26.

The European Kidney Disease Consortium. "The Polycystic Kidney Disease 1 Gene Encodes a 14 kb Transcript and Lies within a Duplicated Region on Chromosome 16." *Cell* 77 (1994): 881–94.

Evers-Kiebooms, G. "Predictive Testing for Huntington's Disease in Belgium." *Journal of Psychosomatic Obstetrics and Gynaecology* 11 (1990): 61–72.

Evers-Kiebooms, G.; Swerts, A.; Cassiman, J. J.; and Van Den Berghe, H. "The Motivation of At-Risk Individuals and Their Partners in Deciding for or Against Predictive Testing for Huntington's Disease." *Clinical Genetics* 3 (1989): 29–40.

Faden, R. R., and Beauchamp, T. L. *A History and Theory of Informed Consent.* New York and Oxford: Oxford University Press, 1986.

Farrer, L. A. "Suicide and Attempted Suicide in Huntington Disease: Implications for Preclinical Testing of Persons at Risk." *American Journal of Medical Genetics* 24 (1986): 305–11.

FitzGerald, M. G.; MacDonald, D. J.; Krainer, M.; et al. "Germline BRCA1 Mutations in Jewish and Non-Jewish Women with Early-Onset Breast Cancer." *New England Journal of Medicine* 334 (1996): 143–49.

Folstein, S. E. *Huntington's Disease: A Disorder of Families.* Baltimore: Johns Hopkins University Press, 1989.

Folstein, Susan E.; Phillips, John A., III; Meyers, Deborah A.; Chase, Gary A.; Abbott, Margaret H.; Franz, Mary L.; Waber, Pamela G.; and Kazazian, Haig H. "Huntington's Disease: Two Families with Differing Clinical Features Show Linkage to the G8 Probe." *Science* 229 (1985): 776–78.

Ford, D.; Easton, D. F.; Bishop, D. T.; Narod, S. A.; Godgar, D. E.; and the Breast Cancer Linkage Consortium. "Risks of Cancer in BRCA1 Mutation Carriers." *Lancet* 343 (1994): 692–95.

Fox, S.; Block, M.; Fahy, M.; and Hayden, M. R. "Predictive Testing for Huntington Disease: I. Description of a Pilot Project in British Columbia." *American Journal of Medical Genetics* 32 (1989): 211–16.

Frankel, M. S., and Teich, A. H. "Ethical and Legal Issues in Pedigree Research." AAAS Committee on Scientific Freedom and Responsibility and the AAAS-ABA National Conference of Lawyers and Scientists. 1993. Pp. 65–87.

Gabow, P. A. "Autosomal Dominant Polycystic Kidney Disease." *New England Journal of Medicine* 329 (1993): 332–42.

Geller, Lisa N., et al. "Individual, Family, and Social Dimensions of Genetic Discrimination: A Case Study Analysis." *Science and Engineering Ethics* 2 (1996): 71–88.

Gert, Bernard; Bernat, James L.; and Mogielnicki, R. Peter. "Distinguishing between Patients' Refusals and Requests." *Hastings Center Report* 24, 4 (1994): 13–15.

Goldberg, Y. P.; Kremer, B.; Andrew, S. E.; Theilmann, J.; Graham, R. K.; Squitieri, F.; Telenius, H.; Adam, S.; Sajoo, A.; Starr, E.; Heiberg, A.; Wolff, G.; and Hayden, M. R. "Molecular Analysis of New Mutations for Huntington Disease: Intermediate Alleles and Sex of Origin Effects." *Nature Genetics* 5 (1993): 174–79.

Gotkin v. Miller, 514 F.2d 125 [2d Cir. 1975].

Grantham, J. J. "Pathogenesis of Renal Cysts in Dominantly Inherited Polycystic Kidney Disease." *Contributions to Nephrology* 115 (1995): 16–19.

Green, J. H., and Barden, R. C. "The Therapist's Duty to Protect the Public from

Dangerous Patients." *Strategies and Solutions: The Journal of Managed Mental Health Care* 1 (1992): 54–58.

Groden, J.; Thliveris, A.; Samowitz, W.; et al. "Identification and Characterization of the Familial Adenomatous Polyposis Coli Gene." *Cell* 66 (1991): 589–600.

Gusella, James F., and MacDonald, Marcy E. "Huntington's Disease and Repeating Trinucleotides." *New England Journal of Medicine* 330 (1994): 1450–51.

Gusella, James F.; Wexler, Nancy S.; Conneally, P. Michael; Naylor, Susan L.; Anderson, Mary Anne; Tanzi, Rudolph E.; Watkins, Paul C.; Ottina, Kathleen; Wallace, Margaret R.; Sakaguchi, Alan Y.; Young, Anne B.; Shoulson, Ira; Bonilla, Ernesto; and Martin, Joseph B. "A Polymorphic DNA Marker Genetically Linked to Huntington's Disease." *Nature* 306 (1983): 234–38.

Hall, J. M.; Lee, M. K.; Newman, B.; Morrow, J. E.; Anderson, L. A.; Huey, B.; and King, M. C. "Linkage of Early-Onset Familial Breast Cancer to Chromosome 17q21." *Science* 250 (1990): 1684–89.

Hannig, V. L.; Hopkins, J. R.; Johnson, H. K.; Phillips, J. A., III; and Reeders, S. T. "Presymptomatic Testing for Adult Onset Polycystic Kidney Disease in At-Risk Kidney Transplant Donors." *American Journal of Medical Genetics* 40 (1991): 425–28.

Harper, Peter. "Ethical Issues in Genetic Testing for Huntington's Disease: Lessons for the Study of Familial Cancers." *Disease Markers* 10 (1992): 189–93.

Harper, P. S. "The Natural History of Huntington Disease." In P. S. Harper, ed. *Huntington's Disease*. London: W. B. Saunders Company, Ltd., 1991, pp. 127–39.

Harper, P., and Sarafazi, M. "Genetic Prediction and Family Structure in Huntington's Chorea." *British Medical Journal* 290 (1985): 1929–31.

Harper, Peter S., and Clarke, Angus. "Should We Test Children for 'Adult' Genetic Diseases?" *Lancet* (1990): 1205–6.

Hayden, M. R. *Huntington's Chorea*. New York: Springer-Verlag, 1981.

Hayden, Michael, et al. "Improved Predictive Testing for Huntington Disease by Using Three Linked DNA Markers." *American Journal of Human Genetics* 43 (1988): 689–94.

Hayden, M. R.; Soles, J. A.; and Ward, R. H. "Age of Onset in Siblings of Persons with Juvenile Huntington Disease." *Clinical Genetics* 28 (1985): 100–105.

Hayes, Catherine V. "Genetic Testing for Huntington's Disease: A Family Issue." *New England Journal of Medicine* 327 (1992): 1449–51.

Heimler, Audrey, and Zanko, Andrea. "Huntington Disease: A Case Study Describing the Complexities and Nuances of Predictive Testing of Monozygotic Twins." *Journal of Genetic Counseling* 4, 2 (1995): 125–37.

Hoskins, K. F.; Stopfer, J. E.; Calzone, K. A.; et al. "Assessment and Counseling for Women with a Family History of Breast Cancer." *Journal of the American Medical Association* 273 (1995): 577–85.

Huggins, Marlene; Bloch, Maurice; Wiggins, Sandi; Adam, Shelin; Suchowersky, Oksana; Trew, Michael; Klimek, MaryLou; Greenberg, Cheryl R.; Eleff, Michael; Thompson, Louise P.; Knight, Julie; MacLeod, Patrick; Girard,

Kathleen; Theilmann, Jane; Hedrick, Amy; and Hayden, Michael R. "Predictive Testing for Huntington Disease in Canada: Adverse Effects and Unexpected Results in Those Receiving a Decreased Risk." *American Journal of Medical Genetics* 42 (1992): 508–15.

Hughes, J.; Ward, C. J.; Peral, B.; et al. "The Polycystic Kidney Disease 1 (PKD1) Gene Encodes a Novel Protein with Multiple Cell Recognition Domains." *Nature Genetics* 10 (1995): 151–60.

Huntington Study Group. Meeting discussion, Baltimore, December 2–4, 1994.

Huntington's Disease Collaborative Research Group. "A Novel Gene Containing a Trinucleotide Repeat That is Expanded and Unstable on Huntington's Disease Chromosomes." *Cell* (1993): 971–83.

Huntington's Disease Society of America. *Guidelines for Predictive Testing for Huntington's Disease*. New York: Huntington's Disease Society of America, 1989.

Huntington's Disease Society of America, Inc. *Guidelines for Genetic Testing for Huntington's Disease*. New York: Huntington's Disease Society of America, Inc., 1994.

Indiana Code Annotated sec. 27-1-12-6(a)(3) (West 1993).

International Huntington Association and World Federation of Neurology. "Ethical Issues Policy Statement on Huntington's Disease Molecular Genetics Predictive Test." *Journal of Medical Genetics* 27 (1990): 34–38.

International Huntington Association and World Federation of Neurology. "Guidelines for the Molecular Genetics Predictive Test in Huntington's Disease." *Neurology* 44 (1994): 1533–36.

International Polycystic Kidney Disease Consortium. "Polycystic Kidney Disease: The Complete Structure of the PKD1 Gene and Its Protein." *Cell* 81 (1995): 289–98.

Jonsen, Albert R., and Toulmin, Stephen. *The Abuse of Casuistry: A History of Moral Reasoning*. Berkeley: University of California Press, 1988.

Karjala, Dennis. "A Legal Research Agenda for the Human Genome Initiative." *Jurimetrics* 32, 2 (1992): 121–222.

Kash, K. M.; Holland, J. C.; Halper, M. S.; and Miller, D. G. "Psychological Distress and Surveillance Behaviors of Women with a Family History of Breast Cancer." *Journal of the National Cancer Institute* 84 (1992): 24–30.

Katz, J. *The Silent World of Doctor and Patient*. New York: Free Press, 1984.

Kessler, Seymour. "Invited Essay on the Psychological Aspects of Genetic Counseling. V. Preselection: A Family Coping Strategy in Huntington Disease." *American Journal of Medical Genetics* 31 (1988): 617–21.

Kessler, Seymour; Field, Tracy; Worth, Laura; and Mosbarger, Heidi. "Attitudes of Persons at Risk for Huntington Disease toward Predictive Testing." *American Journal of Medical Genetics* 26 (1987): 259–70.

Kimberling, W. J.; Fain, P. R.; Kenyon, J. B.; Goldgar, D.; Sujansky, E.; and Gabow, P. "Linkage Heterogeneity of Autosomal Dominant Kidney Disease." *New England Journal of Medicine* 319 (1988): 913–18.

Kimberling, W. J.; Kumar, S.; Gabow, P. A.; Kenyon, J. B.; Connolly, C. J.; Somlo, S. "ADPKD: Localization of a Second Gene to Chromosome 4q13–q23." *Genomics* 18 (1993): 467–72.

Kremer B.; Goldberg, P.; Andrew, S. E.; Theilmann, J.; Telenius, H.; Zeisler, J.; Squitieri, F.; Lin, B.; Bassett, A.; Almqvist, E.; Bird, T. D.; and Hayden, M. R. "A Worldwide Study of the Huntington's Disease Mutation: The Sensitivity and Specificity of Measuring CAG Repeats." *New England Journal of Medicine* 330 (1994): 1401–6.

Langston, A. A.; Malone, K. E.; Thompson, J. D.; Daling, J. R.; and Ostrander, E. A. "BRCA1 Mutations in a Population-Based Sample with Breast Cancer." *New England Journal of Medicine* 334 (1996): 137–42.

Lerman, C.; Daly, M.; et al. "Attitudes about Genetic Testing for Breast-Ovarian Cancer Susceptibility." *Journal of Clinical Oncology* 12 (1994): 843–50.

Lynch, H. T.; Alban, W. A.; Heieck, J. J.; et al. "Genetics, Biomarkers and Control of Breast Cancer: A Review." *Cancer Genetics and Cytogenetics* 13 (1984): 43–92.

Lynch, H. T.; Watson, P.; Conway, T. A.; et al. "DNA Screening for Breast/Ovarian Cancer Susceptibility Based on Linked Markers." *Archives of Internal Medicine* 153 (1993): 1979–87.

MacDonald, M. E.; Barnes, G.; Srinidhi, J.; Duyao, M. P.; Ambrose, C. M.; Myers, R. H.; Gray, J.; Conneally, P. M.; Young, A.; Penney, J.; Shoulson, I.; Hollingsworth, Z.; Koroshetz, W.; Bird, E.; Vonsattel, J. P.; Bonilla, E.; Moscowitz, C.; Penschaszadeh, G.; Brzustowicz, L.; Alvir, J.; Bickham Conde, J.; Cha, J-H.; Dure, L.; Gomez, F.; Ramos-Arroyo, M.; Sanchez-Ramos, J.; Snodgrass, S. R.; de Young, M.; Wexler, N. S.; MacFarlane, H.; Anderson, M. A.; Jenkins, B.; and Gusella, J. F. "Gametic But Not Somatic Instability of CAG Repeat Length in Huntington's Disease." *Journal of Medical Genetics* 30 (1993): 982–86.

Macklin, Ruth. "From 'Moral Issues in Human Genetics: Counseling or Control?' " In Samuel Gorovitz, et al., eds., *Moral Problems in Medicine*, 2nd ed. Englewood Cliffs, N.J.: Prentice-Hall, 1983.

MacMillan, J. C., and Quinn N. P. "Conference Proceedings 15th International World Federation of Neurology Workshop on Huntington's Disease, 31 August–3 September 1993, Boston, Massachusetts, USA." *Journal of Medical Genetics* 30 (1993): 1039–41.

Markel, D. S.; Young, A. B.; and Penney, J. B. "At-Risk Persons' Attitudes towards Presymptomatic and Prenatal Testing of Huntington Disease in Michigan." *American Journal of Medical Genetics* 26 (1987): 295–305.

Mastromauro, Carol; Myers, Richard H.; and Berkman, Barbara. "Attitudes toward Presymptomatic Testing in Huntington Disease." *American Journal of Medical Genetics* 26 (1987): 271–82.

McGlennan, R. C.; Allinson, P. S.; Matthias Hagen, V. L.; Parker, T. L.; Lovell, M. A.; and Kelly, T. E. "Evidence of an Unstable Paternal 27 Repeat Allele in the Huntington Gene Giving Rise to Clinically Overt Huntington Disease in a Patient with the Genotype (17/38)." *American Journal of Human Genetics Supplement* 57 (1995): A246.

Meissen, G. H., and Berchek, R. L. "Intended Use of Predictive Testing by Those at Risk for Huntington Disease." *American Journal of Medical Genetics* 26 (1987): 283–93.

Meissen, Gregory J.; Myers, Richard H.; Mastromauro, Carol A.; Koroshetz,

Walter J.; Klinger, Katherine W.; Farrer, Lindsay A.; Watkins, Patricia A.; Gusella, James F.; Bird, Edward D.; and Martina, Joseph B. "Predictive Testing for Huntington's Disease with Use of a Linked DNA Marker." *New England Journal of Medicine* 318 (1988): 535–42.

Michaud, J.; Russo, P.; Grignon, A.; Dallaire, L.; Bichet, D.; Rosenblatt, D.; Lamothe, E.; and Lambert, M. "Autosomal Dominant Polycystic Kidney Disease in the Fetus." *American Journal of Medical Genetics* 51 (1994): 240–46.

Miki, Y.; Swensen, J.; Shattuck-Eidens, D.; et al. "A Strong Candidate for the Breast and Ovarian Susceptibility Gene, BRCA1." *Science* 266 (1994): 66–71.

Miller, Richard B. *Casuistry and Modern Ethics: A Poetics of Practical Reasoning*. Chicago: University of Chicago Press, 1996.

Misra, V. P.; Baraitser, M.; and Harding, A. E. "Genetic Prediction in Huntington's Disease: What Are the Limitations Imposed by Pedigree Structure?" *Movement Disorders* 3 (1988): 233–36.

Morris, M. J.; Tyler, A.; and Harper, P. S. "Adoption and Genetic Prediction for Huntington's Disease." *Lancet* (November 5, 1988): 1069–70.

Morris, M. J.; Tyler, A.; Lazarous, L.; Meredith, L.; and Harper, P. S. "Problems in Genetic Prediction for Huntington's Disease." *Lancet* (September 9, 1989): 601–3.

Nance, M. A.; Leroy, B. S.; Orr, H. T.; Rish, S. S.; and Heston, L. L. "Protocol for Genetic Testing in Huntington Disease: Three Years of Experience in Minnesota." *American Journal of Medical Genetics* 40 (1991): 518–22.

National Society of Genetic Counselors. "Code of Ethics." *Journal of Genetic Counseling* 1, 1 (1992): 41–43.

Nelkin, Dorothy, and Tancredi, Laurence. *Dangerous Diagnostics: The Social Power of Biological Information*. New York: Basic Books, 1989.

Newman, B.; Austin, M. A.; Lee, M.; and King, M-C. "Inheritance of Human Breast Cancer: Evidence for Autosomal Dominant Transmission in High Risk Families." *Proceedings of the National Academy of Science of the United States of America* 85 (1988): 3044–48.

NIH-DOE Working Group on Ethical, Legal, and Social Implications of Human Genome Research. *Genetic Information and Health Insurance: Report of the Task Force on Genetic Information and Insurance*. Bethesda, Md.: National Center for Human Genome Research, 1993.

Nishisho, I.; Nakamura, Y.; Miyoshi, Y.; et al. "Mutations of Chromosome 5q21 Genes in FAP and Colorectal Cancer Patients." *Science* 253 (1991): 665–78.

Norremolle, A.; Riess, O.; Epplen, J. T.; Fenger, K.; Hasholt, L.; and Sorensen, S. A. "Nucleotide Repeat Elongation in the Huntington Gene in Huntington Disease Patients from 71 Danish Families." *Human Molecular Genetics* 2 (1993): 1475–76.

Novak, R. "Many Mutations May Make Test Difficult." *Science* 226 (1994): 1470.

Parker, S. L.; Tong, T.; Bolden, S.; and Wingo, P. "Cancer Statistics, 1996." *CA: A Cancer Journal for Clinicians* 65 (1996): 5–27.

Peike, S. A.; Kimberling, W. J.; Kenyon, J. B.; and Gabow, P. "Genetic Heterogeneity of Polycystic Kidney Disease: An Estimate of the Proportion of Families Unlinked to Chromosome 16." *American Journal of Human Genetics* 45 Supp. (1989): A58.

Pelias, Mary Z. "Duty to Disclose in Medical Genetics: A Legal Perspective." *American Journal of Medical Genetics* 39 (1991): 347–54.

Peters, D. J. M.; Spruit, L.; Saris, J. J.; Sandkuijl, L. A.; Fossdal, R.; Boersma, J.; van Eijk, R.; Norby, S.; Constantinou-Deltas, C. D.; Pierdes, A.; Brissenden, J. E.; Frants, R. R.; van Ommen, G-J. B.; and Breuning, M. H. "Chromosome 4 Localization of a Second Gene for Autosomal Dominant Polycystic Kidney Disease." *Nature Genetics* 5 (1993): 359–62.

Petersen, G. "Knowledge of the Adenomatous Polyposis Coli Gene and Its Clinical Application." *Annals of Medicine* 26 (1994): 205–8.

Petersen, G. M.; Slack, J.; and Nakamura, Y. "Screening Guidelines and Premorbid Diagnosis of Familial Adenomatous Polyposis Using Linkage." *Gastroenterology* 100 (1991): 1658–64.

Planned Parenthood v. Casey, 112 S. Ct.2791 (1992).

Poelker v. Doe, 432 U.S. 519 (1977).

Powell, S. M.; Petersen, G. M.; Krush, A. J.; et al. "Molecular Diagnosis of Familial Adenomatous Polyposis." *New England Journal of Medicine* 329 (1992): 234–39.

Powell, S. M.; Zilz, N.; Beazer-Barclay, Y.; et al. "APC Mutations Occur Early during Colorectal Tumorigenesis." *Nature* 359 (1992): 234–37.

Preheim, Elissa. "Adoption Practices." Memorandum dated March 22, 1994, on file at the Poynter Center for the Study of Ethics and American Institutions, Indiana University, Bloomington.

Preheim, Elissa. "Insurance Policy Contestability." Memorandum dated March 31, 1994, on file at the Poynter Center for the Study of Ethics and American Institutions, Indiana University, Bloomington.

President's Commission for the Study of Ethical Problems in Medicine and Biomedical and Behavioral Research. *Making Health Care Decisions: Ethical and Legal Implications of Informed Consent in the Patient-Practitioner Relationship. Vol. 1: Report.* Washington, D.C.: Government Printing Office, 1982. Chapter 3, "Decision-Making Capacity and Voluntariness," pp. 55–68.

President's Commission for the Study of Ethical Problems in Medicine and Biomedical and Behavioral Research. *Screening and Counseling for Genetic Conditions: A Report on the Ethical, Social, and Legal Implications of Genetic Screening, Counseling, and Education Programs.* Washington, D.C.: U.S. Government Printing Office, 1983.

Quaid, K. A.; Brandt, J.; and Folstein, S. E. "The Decision to Be Tested for Huntington Disease." *Journal of the American Medical Association* 257 (1987): 3362.

Quaid, Kimberly A. "Presymptomatic Testing for Huntington Disease in the United States." *American Journal of Human Genetics* 53 (1993): 785–87.

Quaid, Kimberly A. "Presymptomatic Testing for Huntington Disease: Recommendations for Counseling." *Journal of Genetic Counseling* 1, 4 (1992): 277–302.

Quaid, Kimberly A. "Psychological and Ethical Considerations in Screening for Disease." *American Journal of Cardiology* 72 (September 30, 1993): 64D–67D.

Quaid, Kimberly A. "Reply to Sharpe (Letter to the Editor)." *American Journal of Medical Genetics* 49 (1994): 354.

Quaid, Kimberly A., and Morris, Michael. "Reluctance to Undergo Predictive Testing: The Case of Huntington Disease." *American Journal of Medical Genetics* 45 (1993): 41–45.

Reeders, S. T.; Breuning, M. H.; Davies, K. E.; Nicholls, R. D.; Jarman, H. P.; Higgs, D. R.; Pearson, P. L.; and Weatherall, D. J. "A Highly Polymorphic DNA Marker Linked to Adult Polycystic Kidney Disease on Chromosome 16." *Nature* (London) 317 (1985): 542–44.

Resta, Robert G. "The Twisted Helix: An Essay on Genetic Counselors, Eugenics, and Social Responsibility." *Journal of Genetic Counseling* 1, 3 (1992): 227–43.

Rhoads, G. G., et al. "The Safety and Efficacy of Chorionic Villus Sampling for Early Prenatal Diagnosis of Cytogenetic Abnormalities." *New England Journal of Medicine* 320 (1989): 609–17.

Roe v. Wade, 410 U.S. 113 (1973).

Rubinsztein, D. C.; Leggo, J.; Coles, R.; Almqvist, E.; Biancalana, V; Cassimen, J. J.; Chotai, K.; Connarty, M.; Craufurd, D.; Curtis, A.; Curtis, D.; Davidson, M. J.; Differ, A. M.; Dode, C.; Dodge, A.; Frontali, M.; Ranen, N. G.; Stine, O. C.; Sherr, M.; Abbott, M.; Franz, M. L.; Graham, C. A.; Harper, P. S.; Hedreen, J. C.; Jackson, A.; Kaplan, J. C.; Losekoot, M.; MacMillan, J. C.; Morrison, P.; Trottier, Y.; Novelletto, A.; Simpson, S. A.; Theilmann, J.; Whittaker, J. L.; Folstein, S. E.; Ross, C. A.; and Hayden, M. R. "Phenotypic Characterization of Individuals with 30–40 CAG Repeats in the Huntington Disease (HD) Gene Reveals HD Cases with 36 Repeats and Apparently Normal Elderly Individuals with 36–39 Repeats." *American Journal of Human Genetics* 59 (1996): 16–22.

Schoenfeld, Miriam; Myers, Richard H.; Cupples, Adrienne; Berkman, Barbara; Sax, Daniel S.; and Clark, Eleanor. "Increased Rate of Suicide among Patients with Huntington's Disease." *Journal of Neurology, Neurosurgery, and Psychiatry* 47 (1984): 1283–87.

Science 256 (April 24, 1992): 480.

Sharpe, Neil F. "Presymptomatic Testing for Huntington Disease: Is There a Duty to Test Those under the Age of Eighteen Years?" *American Journal of Medical Genetics* 46 (1993): 250–53.

Sharpe, Neil F. "Presymptomatic Testing for Huntington Disease: Reply to Quaid." *American Journal of Medical Genetics* 46 (1994): 355–56.

Smurl, James F., and Weaver, David D. "Presymptomatic Testing for Huntington Chorea: Guidelines for Moral and Social Accountability." *American Journal of Medical Genetics* 26 (1987): 247–57.

Snell, R. G.; MacMillan, J. C.; Cheadle, J. P.; et al. "Relationship between Trinucleotide Repeat Expansion and Phenotypic Variation in Huntington's Disease." *Nature Genetics* 4 (1993): 393–97.

Suchowersky, O. "Gilles de la Tourette Syndrome." *Canadian Journal of Neurological Sciences* 21 (1994): 48–52.

Tarasoff v. University of California Board of Regents, 551 P.2d 334 (Cal 1976).

Telenius, H.; Kremer, B.; Goldberg, Y. P.; Theilmann, J.; Andrew, S. E; Zeisler, J.; Adam, S.; Greenberg, C.; Ives, E. J.; Clarke, L. A.; and Hayden, M. R. "Somatic and Gonadal Mosaicism of the Huntington Disease Gene CAG Repeat in Brain and Sperm." *Nature Genetics* 6 (1994): 409–14.

Tibben, A.; Vegter–van der Vlis, M.; Niermeijer, M. F.; Van der Kamp, J. J. P.; Roos, R. A. C.; Roojimans, H. G. M.; Frets, P. G.; and Verhage, F. "Testing for Huntington's Disease with Support for All Parties." *Lancet* 335 (1990): 553.

Tibben, A.; Vegter–van der Vlis, M.; Skraastad, M. I.; Frets, P.; Vanderkamp, J. J. P.; Niermeijer, M. F.; van Ommen, G. B.; Roos, R. A. C.; Roojimans, H. G. M.; Stronks, D.; Verhage, F. "DNA-testing for Huntington Disease in the Netherlands: A Retrospective Study on Psychosocial Effects." *American Journal of Medical Genetics* 44 (1992): 94–99.

Turner, D. R.; Haan, E. A.; Jacka, E.; Kalucy, R. S.; Burns, R. J.; Willoughby, J. O.; and Crabb, R. "Prenatal and Adult Presymptomatic Testing for Huntington's Disease." *Medical Journal of Australia* 148 (1988): 567–73.

Wasmuth, J. J.; Hewitt, J.; Smith, B.; Allard, D.; Haines, J. L.; Skarecky, D.; Partlow, E.; and Hayden, M. R. "A Highly Polymorphic Locus Very Tightly Linked to the Huntington's Disease Gene." *Nature* 332 (1988): 734–36.

Wertz, D. C.; Fletcher, J. C.; and Mulvihill, J. J. "Medical Geneticists Confront Ethical Dilemmas: Cross-Cultural Comparisons among 18 Nations." *American Journal of Genetics* 46 (1990): 1200–1213.

Wertz, Dorothy C.; Fanos, Joanna H.; and Reilly, Philip R. "Genetic Testing for Children and Adolescents: Who Decides?" *Journal of the American Medical Association* 272 (1994): 875–81.

Wertz, Dorothy C., and Fletcher, John C. "Ethics and Medical Genetics in the United States: A National Survey." *American Journal of Medical Genetics* 29 (1988): 815–27.

Wertz, Dorothy C., and Fletcher, John C. "Fatal Knowledge? Prenatal Diagnosis and Sex Selection." *Hastings Center Report* (May–June 1989a): 21–27.

Wertz, Dorothy C., and Fletcher, John C. "Privacy and Disclosure in Medical Genetics Examined in an Ethics of Care." *Bioethics* 5 (1989b): 212–31.

Wexler, Alice. *Mapping Fate.* New York: Random House, 1995.

Wexler, Nancy. "Clairvoyance and Caution: Repercussions from the Human Genome Project." In Daniel J. Kevles and Leroy Hood, eds., *The Code of Codes: Scientific and Social Issues in the Human Genome Project.* Cambridge, Mass.: Harvard University Press, 1992.

Whaley, W. L.; Michiels, F.; MacDonald, M. E.; Romano, D.; Zimmer, M.; Smith, B.; Leavitt, J.; Bucan, M.; Haines, J. L.; Gilliam, T. C.; Zehetner, G.; Smith, C.; Cantor, C. R.; Frischauf, A. M.; Wasmuth, J. J.; Lehrach, H.; and Gusella, J. F. "Mapping of *D4S98/S114/S113* Confines the Huntington's Defect to a Reduced Physical Region at the Telomere of Chromosome 4." *Nucleic Acids Research* 16 (1988): 11769–80.

Wiggins, Sandi; Whyte, Patti; Huggins, Marlene; Adam, Shelin; Theilmann, Jane; Bloch, Maurice; Sheps, Samuel B.; Schechter, Martin T.; and Hayden, Michael R. "The Psychological Consequences of Predictive Testing for Huntington's Disease." *New England Journal of Medicine* 327 (1992): 1402–5.

Wooster, R.; Bignil, G.; Lancaster, J.; Swift, S.; Seal, S.; et al. "Identification of the Breast Cancer Susceptibility Gene BRCA2." *Nature* 378 (1995): 789–91.

Youngman, S.; Shaw D. J.; Bucan, M.; Zimmer, M.; MacDonald, M.; Gilliam, C.; Smith, B.; Wasmuth, J.; Gusella, J., Frischauf, A.; Learch, H.; and Harper, P. S. "D4S90 (D5), a DNA Segment in Close Proximity to Huntington's Disease, Is the Most Terminally Located Probe on the Short Arm of Chromosome 4." *American Journal of Human Genetics* (1988) 43: Abstract 651.

Contributors

Roger B. Dworkin is the Robert H. McKinney Professor of Law at Indiana University School of Law–Bloomington and Nelson Poynter Scholar and Director of Medical Studies at Indiana University's Poynter Center for the Study of Ethics and American Institutions. Dworkin, who has previously served as Professor of Biomedical History at the University of Washington School of Medicine, is an expert on the relationship between law and the biomedical sciences. He is the author of *Limits: The Role of the Law in Bioethical Decision Making,* and numerous articles in the field as well as the coauthor of a leading casebook on law and medicine.

Gregory P. Gramelspacher, M.D., is the founder and Director of the Program in Medical Ethics, Indiana University School of Medicine. He is a general internist with research interests in the areas of death and dying, advance directives, and ethical implications of the human genome project.

Judith A. Granbois joined the staff of the Poynter Center for the Study of Ethics and American Institutions in 1980. She has taught writing and ethics courses at Indiana University and is the coauthor of articles on various topics in biomedical ethics.

Dr. Kimberly A. Quaid is Clinical Associate Professor of Medical and Molecular Genetics and Psychiatry at the Indiana University School of Medicine, where she is also Director of the Predictive Testing Program and Co-Director of the Genetic Counseling Program. Dr. Quaid coordinated one of the first programs in the country to offer predictive testing for Huntington disease at Johns Hopkins Hospital. She works with families at risk for Huntington disease, Gerstmann-Straussler-Scheinker disease, and Alzheimer disease, both in providing education and testing to patients and their families as well as in doing research on the clinical outcomes of testing. She is internationally recognized for her work in the development of ethically sound protocols for genetic testing. She has published numerous journal articles and is author of "Implications of Susceptibility Testing with Apolipoprotein E," in Stephen G. Post, ed., *Ethics, Genetics and Alzheimer Disease.*

David H. Smith is Professor of Religious Studies at Indiana University and Director of the Poynter Center for the Study of Ethics and American Institutions. He is a founding member of the Hospice of Bloomington and the Association for Practical and Professional Ethics. His publications include *Entrusted: The Moral Responsibilities of Trusteeship* and *Health and Medicine in the Anglican Tradition: Conscience, Community, and Compromise.*

Dr. Gail H. Vance is Assistant Professor in the Department of Medical and Molecular Genetics. Dr. Vance joined the Indiana University School of Medicine faculty in 1992, after completing fellowships in clinical genetics and cytogenetics. Dr. Vance is board-certified in Pediatrics (American Board of Pediatrics, 1990), Clinical Pathology (American Board of Pathology, 1989), and Medical Genetics and Clinical Cytogenetics (American Board of Genetics, 1993). Dr. Vance developed the Indiana Familial Cancer Program in the Department of Medical and Molecular Genetics in 1993 to provide genetic counseling and genetic testing to individuals with a high risk for the development of cancer. She is also Assistant Director of the Cytogenetic Laboratory.

Index

Abortion, 1, 23, 25, 42–44, 161–62; laboratory policies on, 90–93
Adam, S., 15
Adoption, 76–79
ADPKD. *See* Autosomal dominant polycystic kidney disease, presymptomatic testing for
Alcoholism, 94, 96, 97
Alper, J. S., 66
American Cancer Society, 17
American Society of Human Genetics/ American College of Medical Genetics, 87–88
Americans with Disabilities Act (ADA), 66
Andrew, S. E., 13, 51
Andrews, Lori B., 47
Anonymous testing, 11–12, 117–20. *See also* Secret testing
Arras, John D., 28
Autonomy, 22, 29, 95
Autosomal dominant diseases, 5–7
Autosomal dominant polycystic kidney disease (ADPKD), presymptomatic testing for, 1, 6, 16–17; of children, 80–83, 165; disclosing results to consultand's adult children, 46–49; disclosing results to potential organ donors, 106–108

Bear, J. C., 16
Benjamin, C. M., 51
Best, Billy, 86
Bloch, Maurice, 12, 91, 95, 102, 112
Brandt, Jason, 12, 13, 95, 102
BRCA1, 17–18
Breast cancer, familial, 7–8, 17–18; disclosure of test results to consultand's parent, 58–61; refusal of test results from

research projects, 39–41, 158–60; psychological impact of testing for, 59–61
Bulow, S., 15

Canadian Collaborative Group, 12
Case studies, 2–7; case selection method, 4–5; Huntington disease as paradigm for, 5–6, 7 8; ordered presentation of, 6–7
Caskey, C. T., 81
Castilla, L. H., 58
Chapman, Marguerite A., 95, 112
Children: ADPKD testing of, 80–83, 165; consultand's refusal to inform adult children, 1, 46–49; disclosing parent's status to adult children, 52; FAP testing of, 84–86, 165; HD testing of, 7, 72–79, 87–89, 91, 163–66; "mature minor" rule for testing of, 82; preselection of, 74, 81; unconceived, 22, 44. *See also* Fetuses, testing of
Clarke, Angus, 88
Clinical Genetics Society (U.K.), 85
Codori, A. M., 13
Collins, F. S., 17
Confidentiality, breaches of, 7, 144–48; disclosing ADPKD test results to consultand's adult children, 46–49; disclosing BRCA1 test results to at-risk family members, 58–61; disclosing HD test results to employers, 62–67, 147; disclosures for public safety, 62–67, 126–28, 145
Conneally, P. M., 8, 9
Corson, Virginia, 91
Counseling. *See* Genetic counseling
Crandall, B., 23

Davies, F., 16
DeGrazia, David, 95, 104
Denial of testing, 94–101, 149–50
Depression, 94, 96, 102–105
Disclosure: of ADPKD results to potential
    organ donors, 106–108; to consultand's
    relatives, 1, 46–49, 58–61, 146; forced
    disclosure to consultands, 31–32, 39–
    41; and others' preferences not to know
    results, 22–28, 42–45, 155–57; refusal
    of, 29–32, 151–54; of research project
    test results, 126–28, 158–60. *See also*
    Confidentiality, breaches of
Discrimination, 2, 66
Duyao, M., 13, 51

Easton, D. F., 17, 58
Emanuel, Ezekiel J., 104
Employers, disclosure to, 62–67, 147
Equal Employment Opportunity Commis-
    sion Compliance Manual, 66
Eugenics, 23
European Polycystic Kidney Disease Con-
    sortium, 81
Evers-Kiebooms, G., 74

Faden, R. R., 103, 107
Familial adenomatous polyposis (FAP),
    presymptomatic testing for, 6, 15–16,
    84–85; of children, 84–86, 165
FAP. *See* Familial adenomatous polyposis,
    presymptomatic testing for
Farrer, L. A., 44, 102
Fetuses, testing of, 1, 23, 25; laboratory
    policy on termination, 90–93; parent
    disagreement in, 42–45
FitzGerald, M. G., 17
Folstein, Susan E., 8, 9
Ford, D., 17, 59
Foster children, testing of, 76–79
Fox, S., 102
Frankel, M. S., 108

Gabow, P. A., 16
Gardner syndrome. *See* Familial adenoma-
    tous polyposis, presymptomatic testing
    for
Gene therapy, 1
Genetic counseling, 2, 7; of anonymous
    consultands, 117–20; appropriate infor-
    mation in, 137–38; disclosing results to
    consultand's family members, 1, 46–49,

53–61; and family competing interests,
    24–25, 42–45; forcing test results on
    consultands, 31–32, 39–41; full range
    of options provided in, 25, 132–35,
    137–38; and improperly obtained pater-
    nity information, 123–25; on insurance
    coverage, 70–71, 118–19; moral educa-
    tion model of, 28; negotiated directive
    model of, 28; nondirective counseling,
    12, 25, 135; and others' preferences not
    to know results, 22–28, 42–45, 155–
    57; and postponement or denial of test-
    ing, 94–101, 149–50; of potential or-
    gan donors, 106–108; pre- vs. posttest
    counseling, 114, 139–41; professional
    values in, 12, 131–36; public safety con-
    cerns in, 62–67, 126–28; on research
    project test results, 39–41, 126–28,
    158–60; for retesting, 37–38; on secret
    linkage testing, 109–12; withholding
    test results by, 133–34
Genetic diseases, presymptomatic testing
    for, 1–2; case study approach to, 2–7.
    See also Autosomal dominant polycystic
    kidney disease; Breast cancer, familial;
    Familial adenomatous polyposis; Hunt-
    ington disease
Gert, Bernard, 95
Goldberg, Y. P., 51
Gotkin v. Miller, 55
Grantham, J. J., 16
Green, J. H., 64
Gusella, James F., 8, 13

Hall, J. M., 17, 58
Hannig, V. L., 16
Haplotype information, 115–16
Harper, Peter, 8, 9, 72
Hayden, Michael R., 8, 30, 88, 102
Hayes, Catherine, 111
HD. *See* Huntington disease, presympto-
    matic testing for
Heimler, Audrey, 25
Hereditary Disease Foundation work-
    shop, 10
Hoskins, K. F., 59
Huggins, Marlene, 12, 30, 31, 40, 74, 95,
    102, 112
Hughes, J., 16
Human Genome Project, 8, 149
Huntington disease (HD), presympto-
    matic testing for, 1; anonymous testing,

117–20; CAG repeat ranges, 13–14, 50–52, 53; of children, 72–79, 87–89, 91, 163–66; compared to diagnosis confirmation, 88; data on demand for, 30; direct testing, 14–15, 119; direct testing as follow-up to inaccurate linkage testing, 33–37; forcing test results on consultands, 31–32; guidelines for testing, 10–12; haplotype information in, 115–16; from improperly obtained paternity information, 123–25; insurance ramifications for, 68–71, 118–19; linkage test for, 8–10; local emotional support during, 102–105; neurologist requests for confirmatory testing, 50–53; as paradigm for case studies, 5–6, 7–8; parent-adult child conflicts in, 26–28; parent disagreement in prenatal testing, 42–45; possible future uses of information, 158–60; postponement or denial of, 94–101, 149–50; protocols for, 102–105, 113–14, 142–43; psychological impact of testing, 12–13, 30–31, 102–105; public safety concerns in, 62–67, 126–28; refusal of test results, 29–32, 151–54; of samples acquired without consent, 121–22; secret linkage testing, 109–12; twins' competing interests in, 21–25; uncertain results from, 50–52
Huntington Study Group, 51
Huntington's Disease Collaborative Research Group, 13
Huntington's Disease Society of America (HDSA) guidelines for testing, 10–12; on adverse emotional responses, 103–104; on informed consent requirements, 100; on postponement or denial of testing, 96, 104; on psychological evaluations in testing protocols, 104–105; on testing of children, 72, 87

Informed consent, 98–99, 107, 121–22, 138
Insurance companies, 118–19; life insurance companies, 68–71
Interests: of consultands, 7, 22; of fetuses, 43–44; of insurance companies, 68–71; of society, 22–23, 62–67; of spouses, 42–45, 47; twins' competing interests, 21–25; of unconceived children, 22
International Huntington Association and World Federation of Neurology

(IHA-WFN) guidelines on testing, 11–12, 96–97, 104–105
International Polycystic Kidney Disease Consortium, 16

Job performance, risks to, 62–67
Johns Hopkins Hospital, 10, 13

Karjala, Dennis, 69, 70, 71
Kash, K. M., 39
Katz, J., 103
Kessler, Seymour, 30, 81
Kimberling, W. J., 16, 80
King, Mary Claire, 17
Kremer, B., 13–14, 53

Laboratory policies on refusing tests, 90–93
Langston, A. A., 17
Lerman, C., 60–61
Life insurance, 68–71
Lynch, H. T., 11, 58

MacDonald, M. E., 51
MacMillan, J. C., 13
Markel, D. S., 30
Mastectomy, prophylactic, 39–41
Mastromauro, Carol, 30
McGlennan, R. C., 13
Medical Information Bureau (MIB), 69
Meissen, G. H., 30
Meissen, Gregory J., 12, 95, 102
Mental disorders, 94–97
Michaud, J., 80
Miki, Y., 17, 58
Misra, V. P., 9
Morris, M. J., 78

Nance, M. A., 12
Nelkin, Dorothy, 69
Newmann, B., 58
Nishisho, I., 15
Nondisclosing prenatal testing, 23, 25, 42, 123–25
Norremolle, A., 13
Novak, R., 58

Organ donors, 106–108
Ovarian cancer, 17, 39, 59

Parents: in conflict over fetal testing, 42–45; refusal of involvement in adult chil-

dren's testing, 26–28; rights and duties of, 26, 42; role of in testing of minor children, 72–75, 80–83; withholding of information from, 53–56, 58–61
Pedigree records, 123–25
Peike, S. A., 16
Pelias, Mary Z., 103
Peters, D. J. M., 80
Petersen, G., 15–16
Planned Parenthood v. Casey, 42
Poelker v. Doe, 42
Powell, S. M., 15, 16, 85
Preheim, Elissa, 69, 77, 78
Preselection, 74, 81
President's Commission for the Study of Ethical Problems in Medicine and Biomedical and Behavioral Research, 48, 63, 99
Protocols, testing, 7, 102–105, 113–14, 142–43
Psychiatric evaluations, 102–105
Public safety, 62–67, 126–28, 145

Quaid, Kimberly A., 12, 30, 31, 47, 72, 74, 91, 95

Reeders, S. T., 16, 80
Renal transplantation, 106–108
Reproductive choices, 7, 22, 161–62. *See also* Abortion
Research projects: disclosure of test results from, 126–28, 158–60; refusal of test results from, 39–41, 158–60
Resta, Robert G., 92
Retardation in consultands, 98–101
Rhoads, G. G., 23
Risks: knowledge of, 49, 60–61; to public safety, 62–67, 126–28, 145; uncertain, 50–52. *See also* Disclosure
Roe v. Wade, 42

Schoenfeld, Miriam, 44, 102
Secret testing, 109–12. *See also* Anonymous testing
Sex selection, prenatal testing for, 92
Sharpe, Neil F., 72, 73, 91
Siblings: informed choice approach for, 56–57; twins' competing interests, 21–25

Skolnick, Mark, 17
Snell, R. G., 51
Spouses: disagreement over fetal testing, 42–45
Suchowersky, O., 88, 89
Suicide, 44, 96, 102, 103

Tarasoff v. University of California Board of Regents, 62, 63–64
Telenius, H., 51
Testing, presymptomatic, 1–2; anonymous testing, 11–12, 117–20; case study approach to, 2–7; of children, 7, 72–88, 91, 163–66; local emotional support during, 102–105; possible future uses of information, 158–60; of potential organ donors, 106–108; protocols for, 7, 102–105, 113–14, 142–43; family conflicts in, 22–28; forcing test results on consultands, 31–32; laboratory policies on refusing tests, 90–93; postponement or denial of, 94–101, 149–50; prenatal testing, 23, 25, 42–45, 90–93, 123–25; psychological impact of testing, 12–13, 30–31, 59–61, 102–105; refusal of results, 29–32, 151–54; of samples acquired without consent, 121–22; secret testing, 109–12; withholding of information from family members, 53–61
Tibben, A., 13
Tourette's syndrome, 87, 88, 89
Twins: conflict over disclosure, 1, 21–25

Wasmuth, J. J., 9, 30
Wertz, Dorothy C., 47, 49
Wexler, Alice, 4–5
Wexler, Milton, 10
Wexler, Nancy, 47
Whaley, W. L., 9
Wiggins, Sandi, 12, 30, 112
Withholding of test results: by consultand from relatives, 1, 53–61; from consultands, 133–34
Wooster, R., 17

Youngman, S., 9

ADX-1434

10/4/00

Armstrong

RB

155.6

E 27

1998